LONNIE BARBACH

For Yourself

Dr. Lonnie Barbach received her M.A. and Ph.D. in clinical social psychology from the Wright Institute in Berkeley, California. She is now on the clinical faculty of the University of California Medical School in San Francisco and also has a private practice. Among her several bestselling books on sex and relationships are *For Each Other, Pleasures, The Erotic Edge*, *The Pause,* and *Going the Distance,* her book with her partner David Geisinger, Ph.D. They live in Mill Valley, California, with their daughter, Tess.

For
Yourself

For Yourself

THE FULFILLMENT
OF FEMALE SEXUALITY

LONNIE BARBACH, Ph.D.

ANCHOR BOOKS
A DIVISION OF RANDOM HOUSE, INC.
NEW YORK

SECOND ANCHOR BOOKS EDITION, MAY 2002

Copyright © 1975, 2000 by Lonnie Garfield Barbach

All rights reserved under International and Pan-American Copyright
Conventions. Published in the United States by Anchor Books,
a division of Random House, Inc., New York, and simultaneously in
Canada by Random House of Canada Limited, Toronto. Originally
published in hardcover in the United States by Doubleday, a division
of Random House, Inc., New York, in 1975. A revised edition was
published in softcover by Signet, an imprint of New American Library,
a division of Penguin Putnam, Inc., New York, in 2000.

Anchor Books and colophon are registered trademarks
of Random House, Inc.

Library of Congress Cataloging-in-Publication Data
Barbach, Lonnie Garfield, 1946–
For yourself : the fulfillment of female sexuality / Lonnie Garfield
Barbach.
   p.   cm.
Includes bibliographical references and index.
ISBN 0-385-11245-9 (trade paper)
1. Sex instruction for women.   2. Women—Sexual behavior.
3. Female orgasm.   4. Masturbation.   I. Title.
HQ46 .B23 1990
613.9'6'082—dc 20
90040476

www.anchorbooks.com

Printed in the United States of America
40   39   38   37   36   35

*In memory of Jay Mann,
who helped launch this book
and with it, my career*

Acknowledgments

My most sincere thanks to my secretary Dianne Cooper, who interpreted my hieroglyphics, to my editor, Kate Medina, who translated them into English, to Dr. Bernie Zilbergeld, Karen Jacobs, and especially Dr. Jay Mann, who devoted time and energy to reading the manuscript, and to Drummond Pike for seeing the process through. I could not have written the book without their help.

I would also like to thank Nancy Carlsen, B. K. Moran, Rebecca Black, Dr. Lynnette Beall, Mary Anne Ver Steege, Toni Ayres, Maggi Rubenstein, June Stanbaugh, Carolyn Smith, Myesha Jenkins, Chuck Jenkins, Marlene Braverman, and my other friends and colleagues who contributed information and perspective. And Betty Dodson for the illustration.

Special thanks and appreciation to the women in the groups who shared their intimate thoughts and feelings and gave me much of the information on which this book is based.

Contents

Introduction

So you've never had an orgasm, or you don't think you have. Or perhaps you only have had orgasms occasionally, or solely through self-stimulation and not with a partner. Or, maybe you just wish you knew more about female sexuality and orgasm.

Do you sometimes feel that you would be happier if sex were eliminated from your intimate relationships altogether? If so, possibly you feel abnormal in this regard, or like a misfit or not whole as a woman. Or, perhaps you just feel that you are missing something everyone else has enjoyed, a part of life that you'd like to have be a part of yours, too. You probably feel as if you are one of only a few women who have this problem. But the truth is that you are far from alone.

In the course of my work as a psychologist and sex therapist with the University of California Medical Center in San Francisco, I have become acutely aware of the extent of the problem many women have in understanding their sexual natures, and in reaching orgasm. Recent statistics on sexual behavior bear out my impressions. With over 1,600 women participating in their study, Laumann, Gagnon, Michael, and Michaels found that a quarter of the women they surveyed had difficulty reaching orgasm. This is an enormous number—one out of every four women. The numbers were *higher* for women under twenty-four, who conceivably had the least sexual experience, and *lower* for women over forty, who had more sexual experience. Never married and divorced or separated women had more difficulty reaching orgasm than currently married women.[1]

Until recently, traditional psychotherapy viewed the presence of a sexual problem as a symptom of an underlying psychological problem or "neurosis." It fostered the notion that "the only effective treatment for total orgasmic impairment is psychotherapy, because the condition is a psychiatric one. The sexual difficulty is simply a manifestation of a deeper emotional dysfunction."[1] As a result of this perspective, many women have been needlessly worried and have paid large sums of money to psychiatrists, yet still experienced little or no change in sexual responsivity.

Dr. William Masters and Virginia Johnson developed a treatment program specifically designed for couples experiencing sexual difficulties. At the University of California Student Health Service in Berkeley, I worked as a therapist treating couples according to the basic Masters and Johnson technique. In this form of therapy, a woman who is not orgasmic is given treatment with her male partner.

Gradually, however, we began to realize that not only was couple treatment too expensive for many women, but also by its very nature it was unavailable to many people who needed help; it restricted treatment only to those women who had steady sexual partners, and to those women whose steady partners were willing and able to attend the counseling sessions. This meant that a large number of women who wanted and needed help were excluded—women whose partners were unwilling or unable to participate in formal treatment, families who could not afford costly couple treatment, women who did not have a steady partner with whom to attend couple treatment, women in homosexual relationships, or the many women who for various private reasons did not want to involve their partners in the problem.

And so, in order to provide help for more women, regardless of the nature of their intimate relationships, I developed, with Nancy Carlsen, a new kind of group treatment program for women that did not entail working directly with a partner[2]—although a more satisfying sexual relationship with a partner remained a primary goal for most women. The new treatment program borrowed elements from the Masters and Johnson therapy technique,[3] and also from other established sex therapy programs, including the series of exercises developed in 1971 by Drs. Lobitz and LoPiccolo at the University of Oregon.[4] What is distinctive about the program is that we worked with women only, in a group situation, and combined a number of therapeutic techniques.

We called the groups "pre-orgasmic" women's groups. Pre-orgasmic seemed a more appropriate term than non-orgasmic, since we fully expected that a woman who entered the group would be orgasmic before the program ended. Each group met for ten sessions of one hour and a half each, spaced over a period of five weeks. Two female coleaders ran the groups. There were five to seven women in each group who were strangers to each other before the first meeting.

The women ranged in age from eighteen to fifty-five years old and came from a variety of ethnic, racial, regional, and religious backgrounds—although, as it happens, the majority of the women were Caucasian and American born. Some were married, some single, others divorced or separated. Some were students, some housewives, some professionals, and others were unskilled workers—although the majority were from what might be generally termed the middle class. A few women were in homosexual relationships, but most were in heterosexual ones and the language of the book reflects this bias. I believe that most of the concepts and techniques in the forthcoming chapters can be helpful to a majority of women. However, each woman is unique—the nature of her relationships, her personality, her background, and her physiological responsivity color her approach to sex as well as to other aspects of her life. In light of this, a variety of exercises is presented, along with discussion of some common difficulties and obstacles encountered by many of the women with whom I have worked.

In a sense the women who participated in the first group sessions are the real authors of this book. When I started the group treatment program, I was already an experienced sex therapist, but the groups taught me a great deal. I want to thank these women (whose names I have changed in the book to protect their privacy) for sharing their lives in the kind of candid detail that enables me to pass on to you not only information, but also specific examples of real-life situations and problems. I hope their candor helps you to open your own experience so that it satisfies your personal needs and desires more fully. In the words of one group member, Carmen, "I hope very strongly that other women will benefit from this therapy as I did. There is a stage where you cannot hope any longer to manage alone, by yourself. I was there and a lot of women must be there, too. I hope that they can find their way to this kind of treatment."

In the group meetings the women shared stories about their sexual difficulties and confusions, their personal feelings about their sexual concerns. Each woman gained insights into her own difficulties from the shared experiences; and each one gained support from the other women's reflections on the possible sources of their sexual problems.

In addition to attending the group sessions, each woman was expected to do one hour of homework every day. This homework, an adaptation of the nine-step masturbation program of LoPiccolo,[5] is fully outlined in this book. The first homework assignments are directed toward helping the woman get in touch with her own body and sexual feelings. Later in the program, when the woman is comfortably orgasmic through self-stimulation, the partner's participation is included in the homework—and so it is included in this book.

The treatment, then, is a combination of group discussions, physiological information about female anatomy and female sexuality, homework exercises, and individualized instruction. The women returned to the group twice a week with new ideas and stories of progress. They worked together and helped each other. They worked hard; they cried, they laughed, they fumed with anger. But most important they did the exercises that paved the way for fuller orgasmic sexual response.

Since the first group met in November 1972, several hundred women have participated in this type of treatment with phenomenal success. Statistics compiled by the Human Sexuality Program at the University of California Medical Center indicate that 93 percent of the women who entered the program, many of whom had never experienced an orgasm, left five weeks later experiencing orgasm consistently, usually through self-stimulation. Of course, the five-week program could not completely reverse a problem, especially if a woman had experienced it for years. The treatment is based on the premise that the woman will continue the exercises on her own, at home. Generally, within three months after the group sessions were over, more than half the women could experience orgasm with partners. After eight months, the percentage was even higher.

The experiences of a pilot group of seventeen women who

were closely followed for eight months after program participation appear typical. Twelve were consistently orgasmic with
a partner while three others were orgasmic over 25 percent of
the time with a partner. Most, but not all, of the women who
reported orgasms with a partner experienced them during
intercourse. Some experienced them through other forms of
love play.

But achieving orgasm was only part of the change that
occurred. Frequently, the impact of the program positively
altered the women's attitudes and feelings about themselves.
By getting in touch with themselves sexually, the women gradually became more comfortable with their own bodies, more
sure of themselves. Betty summed up the change in her feelings about her physical self this way: "I feel very confident now
about my own body's ability to perform. I have learned to
admire my body and to enjoy it."

The simple act of taking the time each day from a busy
schedule to do the homework exercises, making more time for
themselves and their needs, helped many of the women realize
that they deserved more, and consequently further increased
their feelings of self-worth. Many of them began to realize that
other people were willing to respond positively to their requests
for change. Before their experience in the group, many of the
women just assumed that their requests for change would
be rejected or ignored, and so never attempted even to begin
asking.

Another important outcome of the program was that the
women began to take responsibility for their own sexuality,
taking more initiative, communicating their likes and dislikes
more actively. Sexual assertiveness is essential to orgasm. A
study by D. F. Hurlbert showed that sexually assertive women
reported higher frequencies of orgasm in addition to greater
marital and sexual satisfaction.[6] Interestingly, this assertiveness

and assumption of responsibility spread to other areas of the women's lives as well. Research by Arvalea Nelson indicates that consistently orgasmic women tend to describe themselves as contented, good-natured, insightful, self-confident, independent, realistic, strong, capable, and understanding while non-orgasmic women tend to describe themselves as bitter, despondent, dissatisfied, distrustful, fussy, immature, inhibited, prejudiced, and sulky.[7]

My aim in writing this book is to share what has been learned about female sexuality from the groups at the University of California Medical Center. My hope is that the book will serve some of the same functions that the group and orgasmic treatment did for the women who participated in it. The information is also pertinent for men and women without orgasmic difficulties, who want to extend their sexual awareness, and for male and female therapists and educators.

In the book I will address the female reader directly. I have tried to provide the physiological information, the psychological support, and the exercises to enable you to learn more about your own body and its needs, to realize your own sexual potential, and also to overcome the sexual difficulties you may have.

Since the most frequent complaint from women who are dissatisfied with their sex lives is lack of orgasms, this book is specifically designed to counteract that problem. However, since orgasm is just one enjoyable aspect of sex, the larger purpose of the book is to provide information, permission, and support to enable you to experiment and obtain greater satisfaction and enjoyment out of sex whether or not orgasm occurs.

Although sex is one important aspect, much more than sex is involved in a loving relationship. Learning to be open, to share, to communicate and be intimate in nonsexual ways also takes learning and practice. Since some of the nonsexual relationship aspects are beyond the scope of this book, I suggest you read *Going the Distance: Finding and Keeping Lifelong Love*, a book I wrote with my partner, Dr. David Geisinger.

The chapters of this book, *For Yourself*, will follow the general structure of the group therapy program. By reading about the situations, feelings, and experiences of other women, you may be reassured and given a clearer perspective on your own situation. All of us are comforted by knowing that we are not the only person with certain feelings or difficulties. Misinformation about women's sexuality is rampant, and I hope to replace some of it with more accurate facts. In addition to basic information about female sexuality, and stories from the groups, much of the material in the book is aimed at helping you understand your own body and your own sexual responses. Listening closely to the women in the groups destroyed any lingering belief I may have had that there is one way, or a right way, for a woman to respond sexually. These women changed some of my own attitudes about traditional lovemaking and called into question some of the stereotypes under which I had unwittingly been operating. Possibly you'll discover the same for yourself. Each of us is unique. Although we may have some sexual likes, dislikes, and responses in common, we each have an idiosyncratic sexual pattern that is all our own.[8] Just as each of us knows what diet works best when we want to lose weight, and what will best cheer us up when we are feeling blue, each woman can know her sexual self and be an authority on her own body. Once you understand yourself better, it's easier to communicate your sexual needs to a partner.

It may be necessary to reread certain sections of the book from time to time, and to practice the exercises repeatedly before they become effective; the women in the groups frequently found this necessary. Some of the suggestions and exercises might at first seem startling or extreme, but experience has shown that they work.

Since there is no right or wrong, normal or abnormal way to be sexually stimulated, the book makes no attempt to fit you into a mold. Rather its purpose is to encourage you to explore yourself in order to discover your unique sexual responses, at your own speed and with your own goals in mind. My purpose is to provide information that may help you, and in turn help you advise a daughter or friend.

One of the women in the group, the wife of a minister, confided to me that she had approached the group with trepidation, fearing that her religious beliefs might be questioned or faintly ridiculed by the group, or held responsible for her sexual difficulties. After the group was over, she was delighted to find that her sexual problem had been almost fully resolved with no challenge at all to her religious orientation. It is absolutely possible to change your orgasmic response without changing your whole value system—although some of the more traditional views of what is sometimes considered "normal" sexuality may be called into question.

In order to help you begin to understand your individual responsiveness, the exercises begin with self-sexuality. Our group discussions revealed that it is essential for a woman to get in touch with her own body and understand her individual requirements for orgasm before she can effectively communicate her needs to a partner. The easiest and most effective means of getting in touch with your sexual responses is through masturbation. Although important in itself, masturbation turns out to be a very important stepping stone to a healthier, happier self, and a more satisfying and fulfilling sexual relationship with a partner.

For
Yourself

1: Sex and Orgasm

Did you know that minor surgery can be performed on the inner two thirds of the vagina without an anesthetic?[1] Did you know that orgasms with masturbation are usually subjectively reported and objectively recorded as more intense than those resulting from coitus?[2] Did you know that a number of women experience orgasms without even knowing they are doing so?

Because of the fairly widespread ignorance about female sexuality, orgasm is a concern of many, if not most, women. Since we have grown up in a society which, until recently, prohibited much open and direct discussion of sex, many women were left feeling that their own sexual problems or discomforts were unique. When I first met Betty, she had never had an orgasm and had no idea how to go about achieving one. She felt as if there must be a sort of secret, magical society to which some women belonged, and membership qualified those women to have orgasms; that somehow she had never found out how to become a member of the club. It is easy to understand why Betty felt this way; she could think of no other explanation for why she was not privileged to experience orgasm as other women were.

Until recently, it really was not known exactly what women

experienced sexually. Most of what was believed came from writings by men about women's experiences. If what was described in the sex manuals did not match a woman's own personal experience, she assumed they described the experience of most other women. And the mythical experiences described in such books made many women feel inadequate, abnormal. A woman may have secretly hoped that her responses would someday match up with those detailed in the books. The fact that friends rarely discussed sexual problems frankly only confirmed a woman's fears that she was one of the few people having any difficulty in this area. There was almost no information on the subject from a woman's point of view.

In recent years, through more open communication, and with increased scientific investigations into female sexuality, some solid information has been gathered, and these findings describe the sexual experiences of women more accurately than the old sexual myths used to. Basically, the findings show that most women *do* have trouble having orgasm with intercourse.

The statistics cited in the Introduction which show that approximately a quarter of the sexual encounters that end in orgasm for a male partner do not end in orgasm for a female partner give us something to wonder about. If women are not sexually dysfunctional for biological reasons (and how could so many of us be?) it must mean that the current sexual practices employed by many couples, while meeting the needs of a large majority of men, do not meet the unique needs of women. I think it's fair to assume that scientifically, women have the same biological need and capacity for orgasm as men, and that with individual exploration, couple communication, and valid sexual information, we can become capable of enjoying sex and responding orgasmically as often as we wish.

Why all the fuss about orgasm? Why is it so important and

why does the absence of orgasm cause so much frustration and concern? Orgasm is a very pleasurable feeling. More important, orgasm is the natural and normal release of sexual tension. Sexual tension builds up in women just as it does in men. It builds up not only as the result of sexual encounters, but as the result of normal daily activities: the things we see, hear, touch, and think. It builds up more or less depending upon the individual woman and the experiences of her day. And in most of us, this buildup of tension requires a release which is just as natural a process as the buildup itself. In some of us, tension may dissipate without orgasm, while in other women, a continual, repeated lack of sexual release can cause irritability, frustration, fatigue, or headaches. Stress resulting from sexual or other problems can create body imbalances that may result in vaginal infections and other physical symptoms and gynecological problems.[3] Orgasmic release results in pleasure, relaxation, and a feeling of well-being.

Perhaps the best way to describe it would be in the words of Lydia, who wrote after she began to experience orgasm for the first time: "The atmosphere has to be warm, comfortable. No harsh sounds. The feeling of delicious warmth all over my skin, like being covered with warm velvet. Then I begin to concentrate on increasingly pleasant sensations. I feel like I have something extremely warm and soft in my mouth. Sensations are more and more strong and pleasurable in the clitoral area and begin radiating from there to all parts of me. My heart pounds like crazy. I only breathe when I have to. Every part of me seems to extend from my clitoris: head, throat, feet. Then it happens—deep, warm waves roll over and through me in a beautiful rhythm. I always think 'this is the best *ever*.' And then it stops. I'd like to get past the comparison so it could last forever."

That is a description of what one experience of orgasm was

like for one woman. Other women report different experiences, each as unique as the woman herself.

Orgasm, then, is a natural, normal, healthy process. No woman should be prohibited from experiencing the joy of sexual release in her own individual way. It can be as important and necessary for a woman to enjoy sex as it is for her to enjoy her work, children, environment, food, or recreational activities. It's just another potentially satisfying aspect of life.

A woman should be able to delight in sex not only because her body is designed for sexual pleasure, but because a satisfying sexual relationship helps to create a closer and more fulfilling emotional relationship with another person—a lover in the best sense.

Sex has been, and continues to be, a serious point of contention in many relationships. A woman's failure to respond orgasmically within the sexual relationship frequently becomes a source of conflict for the couple,[4] either directly or indirectly, and it is often difficult for a woman to maintain an enthusiastic attitude toward sex if she is not achieving orgasm most of the time. Clark and Wallin reported that two-thirds of the women who had orgasms all or most of the time enjoyed marital intercourse very much, whereas only one-sixth of those who rarely or never had orgasms did.[5]

A pre-orgasmic woman may come to resent her lover's sexual advances and develop ways to avoid them whenever possible. This in turn can have a stifling effect on her partner's demonstrations of affection, not only in the sexual area, but in other areas of intimacy as well. These unexpressed emotions often emerge—the result of some incident, sexual or otherwise—as destructive forces in the relationship. In most cases, if a close relationship is to continue to grow, sex must be a rewarding experience for both people involved.

Then, too, why should a woman leave a sexual encounter feeling frustrated and angry, sad and disappointed, when open, relaxed lovemaking, which often concludes in orgasm, can be such a joyous and validating experience? Laurie describes her feelings after orgasm as being "like a wave has washed over me leaving me spent and so relaxed I want to turn over and go to sleep . . . a tranquilizer. I want to cuddle up to my husband and rest. Often I will have two or three orgasms. Psychologically this is a real boost. It makes me feel important and very good about myself."

Sex and orgasm, then, are normal human functions, and vital parts of a loving relationship. Moreover, sexual responsiveness is an important part of a woman's self-image. Most of the women I have worked with felt that there must be something basically wrong with them because they did not have orgasms. The women felt vaguely ashamed of themselves, and tried to hide the problem from others—either by not talking about it, or by keeping sexual encounters to a minimum and faking orgasm when they did make love. Connie claimed that her husband separated from her as a result of her sexual unresponsiveness. At the time she entered the group, she had had no sexual relationships since their separation. Because she had never had an orgasm, she felt incomplete as a woman and could not imagine that another man would want her, given this inability. So feeling good about oneself and one's responsivity as a female can be another important reason to have orgasms.

A number of common fears, false expectations, and misinformation seem to prevent many women from realizing their full sexual potential.

The first erroneous belief shared by many women in the therapy program is that sexual behavior comes naturally. A colleague of mine, Thea Lowry, puts it well, "Although sex is perfectly natural, it is not always naturally perfect." Many women don't know how to respond orgasmically and yet they feel they *should* know, since sex is supposed to be a normal animal instinct. So there is a tendency to just wait for it to "happen," for something to click. Unsatisfactory sex comes naturally, but good sex, for both men and women, requires information, practice, communication, and cooperation. Women are not "frigid." The term "frigid" implies numerous negative psychological attributes that have nothing to do with lack of orgasm.

The human brain is the most complex of any species. According to Ford and Beach, "This explains why, in human beings more than other species, sexuality is structured and patterned by learning."[6] Sex is actually less instinctive in the human being. Like any other skill, it needs to be learned and to be practiced. Kinsey found that as the years of marital sexual experience increased, sexual responsivity increased.[7] Margaret Mead found that in the human female the potentiality for orgasm is a cultural factor. If a society considers orgasmic release of the female important, then the essential lovemaking techniques necessary to ensure the woman's orgasm will be learned and practiced. If the female orgasm is considered unimportant, the members of the culture will not practice techniques essential to orgasmic release in the woman; and women are likely to be anorgasmic.[8]

A second erroneous expectation is that the man should be the authority on sex—that the man is responsible for the woman's orgasm. Expecting this to be the case can lead to all sorts of erroneous conclusions. "Maybe it's not love," is one way of dismissing the difficulty. After all, you might feel that if it were really love, you would feel so turned on that you would naturally have orgasms. Because you don't have orgasms, you may assume that your partner must not be "Mr. Right," and you must not really be "in love" with him. Besides, if he really loved you, wouldn't he know how to "give" you an orgasm? Since he doesn't "give" you orgasms, you may conclude that he must not love you enough.

These feelings stem from the misconception that the man should know all there is to know about sex. Most of us have never been given accurate and specific information about sex, but rather have been led to believe that sex is a man's area of expertise. And if a woman is experienced, she is taught that she should remain silent about it. As I think back on it now, I grew up believing men were somehow born with the knowledge about sex, never thinking that they, too, needed to be taught just as I did. Dr. Bernie Zilbergeld, a colleague who leads sex therapy groups for men, reports that many of the men in his program say they would love it if their partners were free in expressing sexual desires. They feel this would relieve them of a heavy burden—they could admit some sexual ignorance and stop straining to seem expert.

Men do not have any magical answers for successful sex and they are not capable of reading a woman's mind to find out what she wants and needs. They need to learn how a woman likes to make love, just as they need to learn how she takes her coffee. Waiting for "Mr. Right" to come along and light your orgasmic fire could take forever. One might go from lover to lover in search of the explosive spark and fail to work on the positive possibilities of any one relationship. Women who have had many lovers expect their solution to come when they find a truly meaningful relationship, while women who are involved in a rewarding and intimate relationship secretly suspect that the answer lies in experiencing a variety of men.

Sally and Rita were in the same women's group. Rita reported having more than fifty different male sex partners and claimed that if only she could find a meaningful and long-term relationship, her orgasmic problem would be solved. Sally, on the other hand, was a virgin when she married, and continued to be very much in love with her husband. She secretly suspected, however, that if she had just had more experience with other lovers, her problem would be over. They each realized, hearing the other talk, that the solution didn't necessarily lie in the number of different lovers, or the intensity of the relationship. Women in intense relationships can be non-orgasmic while others in casual affairs might have little or no difficulty achieving orgasm.

Sometimes looking for the right man is translated into the search for the "magic penis." If you could just find the right penis—a bigger one, a smaller one—or if you could just find an erection that would last long enough, your orgasmic problems would be solved. But the fact is that the size of an erect penis varies only slightly.[9] Moreover, intercourse is only one technique for lovemaking; women can reach orgasm through other kinds of stimulation—oral or manual. So the male partner doesn't even have to have an erection at all to satisfy a woman sexually. The kind of stimulation that suits the specific woman is what counts. This is especially important because no two women respond in exactly the same way sexually. Each individual has her own personal likes, dislikes, and favorite types of stimulation. But, of course, a woman can't tell a partner what she likes, what stimulates her best, if she doesn't know herself. Basically, an understanding of your unique sexual self, sometimes most easily acquired by the process of self-stimulation, can put you in a better position to help your partner learn how to please you.

Another false expectation is that orgasm "should" occur through intercourse alone; women tend to feel sexually "imma-ture," even "neurotic," if they require direct clitoral stimulation to achieve orgasm. They disqualify these orgasms. They want "vaginal" orgasms. They want orgasms the "right" way—that is, during intercourse. We have bought the idea that the vagina is the primary sex organ and that therefore, the only real way to have a "mature" orgasm is through the thrusting of the penis in and out of the vagina.

In reality, the clitoris is the female sex organ. Roughly comparable in sensitivity to the penis, the clitoris serves no other function than that of providing sexual pleasure. The vagina is comparable in sensitivity to the male testicles. Therefore, if instead of sexual intercourse, which directly stimulates the male's most sensitive organ, and only indirectly stimulates the female's most sexually sensitive organ, lovemaking were practiced by a male rubbing the clitoris with his testicles—then women would be orgasmic and men would be in groups for pre-orgasmic treatment!

As Sarah put it when she first came to the group, "If the old thrusting in and out would do it, it would have happened by now. Since it didn't, I'm now ready to try other things."

The physiological fact is that intercourse alone just doesn't seem to provide enough of the right kind of stimulation in the right area to permit many women to become aroused to the point of orgasm. Physiologically, it may not be possible for you to have orgasms through intercourse unless you also receive additional direct clitoral stimulation. As Ann Koedt says, "If certain sexual positions now defined as 'standard' are not mutually conducive to orgasm, they must no longer be defined as standard."[10]

Another common erroneous expectation is that a woman should have her orgasm at the same time her partner does, in one glorious simultaneous climax. I'm certain none of these "shoulds" have been scripted by women. They just don't meet many physiological requirements for female orgasm.

One of the most detrimental of the erroneous beliefs is that sex is not as necessary for women as it is for men. Women are taught that a woman does not need the sexual release that a man does, that a man's sexual needs are greater than a woman's and she must accommodate him. This can produce an unfortunate situation at either extreme. If a woman feels she has no rights of her own, but must accommodate her partner whenever he is sexually interested, she will very likely end up feeling resentful most of the time. Constant sexual availability is not one of the marriage vows. On the other hand, if a woman believes she is not supposed to express herself sexually, she may inhibit her natural desire for fear she will appear unfeminine.

Woman is not asexual. If she is aggressive and assertive sexually it doesn't mean she is masculine. Passivity is not the normal female state. Expressing yourself sexually for yourself and not just for your partner is essential.

Feelings of repulsion and disgust about sex can be a factor inhibiting sexual expression. Sex repulsion is a reaction usually based on early negative messages about sex, some of which may have been perceived unconsciously. The most prevalent basis for repulsion toward sex comes from the erroneous idea that women's genitals are disgusting and dirty and hence sex is disgusting and dirty. As children, our genitals became associated with the organs of excretion, and we grew up feeling that "down there" was an unclean and unacceptable part of our body. Lydia never had an orgasm. She never touched her genitals directly with her hands because she felt her genitals were so repulsive. She found great difficulty in even looking at the area in a mirror, but after doing so was surprised that it was much nicer than she had anticipated. She overcame her negative feelings about her genitals by getting more familiar with them, both visually and tactilely, and soon thereafter could experience orgasms with masturbation. Eve always felt her vagina was extremely dirty and was surprised to learn that the vagina is generally cleaner than the mouth.

Other reasons for developing a repulsion toward sex can come from experiences of sexual contact with adults at an early age—rape and other sexual molestation may cause a young woman to feel dirty or promiscuous, or to find sex repulsive. As a child, Eve had been sexually fondled by her father and her older brother. Her brother, in particular, threatened to physically hurt her if she refused to submit or if she told anyone about it. Quite understandably, Eve could not reconcile the pleasurable sexual feelings with the fact that she was doing something that was considered wrong. When she grew older and married, any sexual feeling would bring up her childhood sexual experiences and the feelings she had spent years trying to forget. It was difficult for Eve to explore her sexuality because she would have preferred to experience no sexual feelings whatsoever. This sort of scenario is surprisingly common. An educated guess places incest at about one million cases per year in the United States.[11] In a 1994 study, 17 percent of women reported that they had been sexually touched when they were children.[12] Old traumas don't die quickly, but gradually Eve is becoming more comfortable with experiencing and expressing her sexual feelings as an adult who has control in her adult sexual relationship.

Another source of inhibition is the fear some women have that they will look ugly while they are having an orgasm and that their partners will be repulsed and find them unattractive. This was a tremendous fear of Carmen's, and after her partner saw her having an orgasm for the first time, she repeatedly asked him if she looked ugly, and if he still loved her. He responded very supportively and told her that she looked beautiful and that he deeply loved her. After having a few more orgasms and still no negative reactions, she was finally convinced he was telling the truth.

The fear of losing control, of fainting, or of screaming while having an orgasm are other common concerns among women who have never experienced orgasm. All the Victorian pornographic novels depict women as fainting or dying away when they have an orgasm. This does not happen in reality. However, the fear of losing consciousness is natural, since at the point of orgasm, there is lessened outside awareness. Carmen became very upset because, as she was about to experience her first orgasm with masturbation, her lover touched her. She had not even been aware that he had entered the room and had neither heard nor seen him because she was so involved in self-stimulation. The intensity of her sexual involvement really distressed her. However, the fact that she could regain control when he touched her helped her to realize that she hadn't lost consciousness, but had only had her attention focused more internally than externally. Carmen was able to overcome this initial upset and have her first orgasm a few days later.

Carol was afraid she would have to grow up and become a responsible woman if she had orgasms. Eve felt that going "all the way" meant having an orgasm. She rationalized that she was really a "good girl" because even though she was having sex, she was not really "going all the way." She could let her sexual feelings go only so far—even though she was married. Leslie was afraid she would do things she thought were immoral if she started experiencing orgasms. Other women, including Janice, were afraid that having an orgasm would change their lives. What did happen when these women began having orgasms after the therapy program? Carol didn't have to grow up any more than she wanted to. Eve was no less virtuous and certainly never became promiscuous. Leslie became a little less conservative, but definitely not immoral or perverted by her standards, and Janice's whole life didn't change. She just felt a little bit better about herself and whole lot better about sex.

Many things cause changes in our lives. Few of us live by a totally regimented routine that never varies. We marry, divorce; have children; our children get older and finally leave home; we change jobs, we move to a new house, and unexpected events cause us to change our plans. But we usually have some measure of control over our life circumstances. A tornado of change doesn't usually uproot us and whirl us around to the degree that we don't recognize our former selves. Changes are generally slow and gradual.

Experiencing orgasms, when you haven't previously, might result in greater enjoyment of sex, a closer, more intimate relationship, and possibly even fewer sexual inhibitions and greater assertiveness in the bedroom. You might note some of these changes, but I doubt that you'll feel so different that you won't recognize yourself or that all your life problems will suddenly appear resolved.

Some women fear that if they become orgasmic with a man that they will be completely dependent upon him and hence more vulnerable. Evelyn never felt she could trust men. She said men could never be counted on, that they will just take off and leave you. She feared that if she became orgasmic with her husband, she would be more vulnerable if he left her because then she would be dependent upon him for orgasms. Objectively this just doesn't make sense, even though the fear is real. If you can have orgasms with one partner, you can probably have them with another or by yourself through masturbation. No one "gives" you orgasms. You are the one in control. You let them happen or shut them off. Furthermore, it's likely you'll be just as vulnerable and hurt if your lover should leave you whether or not you have been having orgasms when you make love.

A real fear that can keep some women from doing anything to solve their sexual problems is the fear of failure. When Harriet joined the group, she didn't believe she could become orgasmic. She said, "If I tried, I'd only fail, and then I'd be *really* miserable." Harriet felt hopeless and helpless. She had created a self-fulfilling prophecy. By deciding ahead of time that she would fail, she never really tried to do anything positive to become orgasmic. The group members pointed out that if she *never* tried to do anything about it, her prophecy *would* come true. She would never become orgasmic. However, if she tried—conscientiously—she would at least have a chance at succeeding.

Harriet eventually did defy her fears, as did all the other women mentioned. It takes time and effort to counteract these fears. It means saying "I'm afraid" and yet pushing beyond.

All of the sexual fears, myths, and erroneous expectations I have described were first mentioned by the pre-orgasmic women with whom I have worked. You may have some of these same fears or, perhaps, different ones. The women in the groups started having orgasms despite their fears, and you can, too; or, if you already are orgasmic but not consistently so, you can build a richer sexual life.

Are any of the points that have been discussed true for you? Are you pre-orgasmic because you're different and hence special if you don't have orgasms? Do you feel that you have been so deprived in your past that it's too late, that you can't make up for all your early deprivations now? It's never too late. Many women begin enjoying sex more as they grow older. Leslie was forty-eight years old before she experienced her first orgasm, and now she's enjoying sex more than she ever has in her life.

Do you think you aren't orgasmic because you're nervous? Or that you feel you are neurotic and have to solve your emotional problems before you can expect your sex life to be satisfying? No one is totally free of emotional hang-ups, but despite psychological difficulties one can enjoy sex and be orgasmic, too. If you think you have to feel totally good about yourself, your life, your job and children before you will be able to experience orgasm, you may be waiting around forever. This is one reason why traditional psychotherapy has never been very successful at curing anorgasmia.[13] Working directly on the mental problems can help to resolve them, and possibly help in sexual areas as well, but it is often more efficient to work directly on the sexual problem if you decide you want to change it. Joan saw a gynecologist because she could not have orgasms. The physician recommended that she undergo psychoanalysis. For two years she worked through her problems with her mother, father, sisters, and brothers, but still never had an orgasm. She started having orgasms only after she came to the women's groups and learned about her sexual anatomy and about masturbation.

Is it because you're too embarrassed to ask for what you want at a particular time; afraid your partner will refuse, get angry, or feel emasculated? Is lovemaking too short and too fast for you?

Would it be a relief if your doctor told you that you couldn't be orgasmic? Would it be easier to accept that you're a physical anomaly? The truth is, you're probably not. According to Helen Kaplan, general *loss of sexual interest* can reflect "underlying debilitating illness, fatigue, depression, or the use and abuse of certain drugs. Fluctuating hormonal states as during the menstrual cycle or in pregnancy or the use of contraceptive medication"[14] do not necessarily affect orgasmic response. Cases of physical disabilities that affect orgasm are exceedingly rare in an otherwise sexually responsive female. Some women who take certain antidepressants, the serotonin re-uptake inhibitors (SSRIs), such as Prozac and Zoloft, find they have difficulty reaching orgasm. However, solutions do exist. One study shows that 120 mg of Ginkgo biloba taken twice a day can mitigate the problem for about 90 percent of the women taking it. Others find that if they switch to Serzone, or some of the other newer medications, the orgasm problem resolves.[15]

In almost all cases, if you have a clitoris, you can be orgasmic if you want to. But what can you do about it? You may be willing to try anything, but you may not know where to begin.

Relearning about your sexuality can be enjoyable but requires time and practice. It means that you have to assume responsibility and be somewhat assertive. Our culture has taught us that a woman should depend on a man to take care of her, which means she can blame him for any mistakes. It's nice to be driven around in a car, but it's also nice to be able to drive yourself so you can go where you want to, when you want to. But to do that, you'd have to assume some responsibility. Many women have been trained into passivity. They've been taught to hold back, or hide their strengths and desires. Lethargy, boredom, and feelings of powerlessness can result from not asserting oneself. The cure is not rest and tranquilizers, or the psychoanalyst's couch, but participation. While it's risky to set out to accomplish something by yourself, for yourself, succeeding can be worth it.

According to Ovid's legend, Zeus and Hera were arguing about which one, man or woman, derived more pleasure from sex. Since Tiresias had been both a man and a woman, they called upon him to settle the argument. To this question, Tiresias quickly responded that women did.[16] Perhaps Tiresias is right; we have no way of really knowing, since we can't switch sexes. However, there is probably no reason why you can't enjoy sex fully and be orgasmic. Look to the wisdom of your body, your feelings and instincts. After you find out what really turns you on, you can change your sexual practices to fit your responses, rather than attempting to react to the things you *think* should turn you on. You'll never really know how your subjective experiences compare to those of another person, but if you are enjoying yourself, it really doesn't matter.

2: Sources of Sexual Confusion

Until recently, most women have accepted male views of female sexuality. Even when these views may have conflicted with a woman's own self-knowledge, she acquiesced or remained silent rather than challenge the authorities who were predominantly male—researchers, writers, doctors, psychologists, religious leaders, and family breadwinners. Furthermore, many women considered themselves inadequate and abnormal if their experiences conflicted with the words of the "authorities."

Freud made the first intensive exploration of the psychological aspects of sexuality and, like many pioneers who approach a totally unknown area, he arrived at some biased conclusions. Freud concluded, ". . . that in the phallic phase of girls the clitoris is the leading erotogenic zone. But it is not, of course, going to remain so. With the change to femininity the clitoris should wholly or in part hand over its sensitivity, and at the same time its importance, to the vagina."[1] In direct contrast to Freud's position, the more recent physiological findings of Masters and Johnson show that no switch in area of responsivity ever occurs and that the clitoral area remains the area most sensitive to sexual stimulation throughout most women's lives.[2]

Until recent years, women who sought the help of doctors for their orgasmic problems often found that their "inadequacy" and "abnormality" were confirmed by their doctors. Members of the medical profession based their judgment of normality mainly on what Freud and others had outlined. Some physicians went so far as to attempt to eliminate the problem by eliminating the clitoris. One theory argued that if the clitoris and its surrounding structures were removed, this area would not interfere with the vagina's sensitivity. Clitoridectomies, as various forms of this operation were called, were sometimes performed on young girls in Europe during the late 1800s to inhibit masturbation, and on young women to prevent unfaithfulness.[3] However, nowhere in the literature do we find recommendations that the penis or testicles be removed to curtail the masturbatory activities of boys, or the adulterous activities of men. One woman who came to the University of California clinic to be treated for orgasmic difficulties had had the hood of her clitoris removed when she was four years old because of "excessive" masturbation—and clitoridectomies are commonplace in some cultures.

Women who today seek help from physicians for orgasmic difficulties will not be given a clitoridectomy, but neither are they always likely to be given accurate information or pertinent advice in the area of sexual functioning. The general lack of accurate knowledge among physicians about sexual functioning is easy to understand if one remembers that sexuality and sexual functioning are largely ignored in the curriculum of most medical schools. Thus, you find yourself seeking help from "authorities," who may in actuality know less about sexuality than you know. They, too, are victims of a culture that subscribes to outdated notions.

Evelyn was married at sixteen and after four years of marriage went to her doctor because she had never experienced an orgasm and felt there might be something medically wrong. Her doctor told her that she did not have orgasms because her sex organs had not quite "matured" yet and that after they did, in a few years or so, she would become orgasmic. This advice was totally inaccurate; female infants as early as four months of age are reported to have experienced orgasm.[4] But Evelyn believed the doctor, and as she waited for this maturing process miraculously to take place, she became less interested in and more resentful about sex. At thirty-five, when she began the group, she was furious at having wasted years before doing something more positive about the problem. One doctor told Judy that she shouldn't concern herself about not having orgasms, that it's not necessary for a woman to have orgasms. When Kim complained to her doctor about not liking sex, he told her to participate because of her husband's needs, because sex was her husband's privilege. One woman was even told by a doctor not to masturbate. He said it was important for her to save all her sexual feelings for her husband—as if masturbation would "use up" her sexual desire.

Sally was a virgin when she married, and when she went to her physician for her premarital exam, he informed her about what to expect with intercourse. He told her it would feel like a steel rod being shoved into her vagina and that it would be very painful. Her reaction was to develop vaginismus and dyspareunia. (Vaginismus is the name given for excessive tightening of the muscle of the vaginal opening. Dyspareunia is the medical term for pain with intercourse.) Since she expected sex to be a painful experience, she tensed her vaginal muscles to help guard against the anticipated hurt. Ironically, her attempt to protect herself from the pain actually caused it.

Most sins perpetrated by doctors in the area of sexuality, however, result more from omission than commission. Some doctors just haven't received the necessary training in sexuality to be able to help patients with sexual problems. Sexual dysfunctions are frequently glossed over, possibly in the hope that if the patient stops worrying, her problem will resolve itself. Certainly, orgasmic dysfunction is not a life-or-death problem, but it is an area of considerable concern to many women. Relieving the overconcern and worry is essential to reversing the situation, but is frequently insufficient in itself.

Western religious and moral upbringing has also been influenced mainly by men, since it is men who hold the positions of authority in most religions. Many organized religions have traditionally regarded sex as intended primarily for procreation. Women are seen alternately as sexually pure—the madonna—or basically carnal with sexual appetites that need to be suppressed—the whore/temptress.[5] This confusion between sexuality and morality has been another source of conflict for many women.

So, it is not surprising that many women enter adult sexuality feeling uneasy, embarrassed, unsure, sinful. In the words of sex therapist Thea Lowry, "Psychologists have put a pathological label [frigid] on women who are unable to do as adults, what they were brought up to be unable to do." Many of us received clear messages while growing up that presented sex as bad, dirty, a subject best avoided. We may have been taught that a nice girl wasn't even supposed to know that such a thing as sex existed, at least not until after she was married. Then, miraculously, sex was supposed to lose all its nasty connotations and become a joyful experience.

In our very early years, before we even knew sex existed, many of us were taught not to explore our bodies "down there," and were reprimanded if our hands wandered in that direction. We may have been given separate washcloths, one for our face and hands, and one for the unmentionable "other place." The message was clear; it must be terribly dirty and disgusting down there. Ironically, Gloria discovered her orgasm precisely as the result of those negative messages. She put that extraordinarily dirty place directly under the faucet of the tub in order to wash it more thoroughly and was pleasantly surprised to find that the pressure of the water created a most intense sensation which culminated in orgasm, although she did not recognize it as such at the time.

Somewhere, either directly or indirectly, many of us got the message that we shouldn't touch our genitals, and so, when we did, we felt ashamed and confused. Boys were praised for handling their penises when they were toilet trained, whereas girls were diverted from direct genital contact. If we allowed our hands to linger on our genitals long enough, we may have experienced the pleasure derived from touching the clitoris. But we never heard anyone else mention these pleasant sensations. As a result, we may have grown up feeling weirdly unique—as though no other girl did such things and felt such things. Feeling that we must be abnormal or immoral, we may have made silent pacts with ourselves that we would touch ourselves just this time and never again; but we were forever breaking this promise to ourselves and to the omniscient God observing us from above. Often, when we did give in, we masturbated as surreptitiously and quickly as possible in an attempt to avoid the feelings of shame and guilt.

Mary grew up with the idea that touching herself "down there" was sinful, if not physically harmful. She did not realize that what she was doing was masturbation and was only vaguely aware that it had anything to do with sex. One day, just before taking a nap, she masturbated. When she awoke, she was ill and was sure that the illness was caused by touching herself before falling asleep even though she had done it many times before with no adverse effects. She was so frightened that she avoided masturbating for months afterward.

The natural curiosity of children includes the desire to explore their own bodies—everywhere—and to explore the bodies of others. In darkened basements with flashlights, out behind the garage, or in the grass among the trees, we furtively and curiously examined each other to see how we were similar or different. "Playing doctor" gave us the thrill of dangerous exploration but also the guilt and fear of being caught—with our pants down, so to speak.

We learned quickly that we shouldn't ask questions about sex or about "that" part of our body which was supposed to remain a mystery to us until marriage. (It is interesting to note that this very area of the body which was so dirty, secret, and shameful, was also purported to be the most sacred gift you could give, unsullied, to your husband on your wedding night.) If we did ask about sex, the embarrassment evidenced by our elders quickly convinced us not to ask again. We had only two avenues for our ignorance—books or miscellaneous information gathered from friends.

The most frequent source of misinformation came from peers who rarely knew any more than we did. We may have gotten the egg and sperm story straight, but how the egg met the sperm remained a mystery. Looking to the written authority to help us out wasn't much better. Of course, the greatest authority was the dictionary, was it not? The dictionary method went something like this: We looked up a word we had already heard, but weren't exactly sure about. For example, the word *intercourse*. The second definition in *Webster's New World Dictionary* states: "Sexual joining of two individuals; coitus; copulation."[6] Well, we already knew that much, but we wanted to know just exactly how this was done. But here are two new words, *coitus* and *copulation*. So we look up *coitus* and the definition is "sexual intercourse."[7] Nothing new on that round! *Copulation* wasn't much help, either. So maybe we persevered and began again with *vagina*: "A sheath or sheath-like structure; specifically, in female mammals, the canal leading from the vulva to the uterus."[8] The only thing we've learned is that we don't know what the vulva or uterus is. And so the search continued in this circuitous and frustrating manner.

Being female and fearing disapproval, we carefully kept our sexual curiosity a secret. We learned the traits of being "feminine," to depend on others and to seek their love. Hence, most of us readily learned to adapt, and not make trouble. To be passive was to be loved. But being passive frequently meant giving up control over one's body: learning to trade tomboy tree climbing, no matter how much we enjoyed it, for being the mother of dolls. Girls were praised for being clean, pretty, and unobtrusive. Boys were expected to be active, to aggressively explore and confront situations head-on, while girls were to be protected, comforted, and cared for. We were considered too delicate to endure the bumps and bruises that exploration inevitably produced. So, trading vigor for prudence, we shaped our behavior to conform to the expectation that males are aggressive while females are restrained. As a result, many of us ended up expecting our male partners to be the active initiators in sex while we remained the passive recipients.

Being passive and striving for love as a measure of self-worth—rather than making an impact upon the world—created some traumatic and almost intolerable situations for many young girls. This passive stance may have made some girls particularly susceptible to molestation or incest, which, if it generates enough fear, shame, or guilt, can result in orgasmic difficulties later in life.

Whether or not we experienced sexual traumas before puberty, the onset of menstruation often caused conflicts and problems. Some women who had been given no information about menstruation recall that they reacted to the first menstrual flow with terror: were they hurt or sick? Even if it was explained ahead of time, the circumstances rarely seemed conducive to open and unembarrassed communication. Some of our mothers handed us books on "growing up" while others merely left books lying around where we were certain to find them. This way of handling the topic opened and closed the subject, all in one motion. We quickly perceived that this wasn't a topic for candid discussion. If Mother actually did discuss "growing up" with us, usually we felt her embarrassment, which was in turn the result of her own sexual upbringing. Even if we did have a solid, communicative relationship with our mothers, we still found ourselves plagued with blood and cramps each month. Ironically, just because we were now "women" and could someday experience the joy of bearing children, we were supposed to have an elated response to something that has been nicknamed the "curse." The prospect of children seemed a slim reward—especially since we would have to wait approximately ten years to collect. Meanwhile, we remained self-conscious about it all.

Angela talked about putting in tampons for the first time. Studying the diagram enclosed in the package merely added to her already considerable confusion about what her body was like inside. She finally found the courage to insert a tampon, in what she hoped was the right place. She was convinced that it ended up being lodged somewhere between her heart and her stomach. Angela's experience was by no means unique. Sadie inserted the tampon, cardboard container and all, and couldn't understand why the product—which advertised itself as being completely unnoticeable when in place—was so painful. Another group member abandoned the use of tampons just a few months after beginning to use them. She explained that they were just too painful to insert. Somewhere she had gotten the idea that the tampon had to be as far inside as possible in order to work properly, so she was putting the cardboard all the way in before releasing the tampon.

Although some of our mothers felt pride when we menstruated, we felt mainly discomfort. Moreover, after explaining menstruation, many of our mothers gave us no further information about sex; they remained embarrassed and we remained curious. Laura actually had intercourse at the age of nineteen without realizing that it was intercourse. A number of women in the groups felt a good deal of anger, especially toward their mothers, for not providing them with the necessary information about sex or for treating sex as a dirty activity, rather than emphasizing its joyous qualities.

Repressive attitudes toward sex, as we know them, are not universal. According to Ford and Beach, "The societies that severely restrict adolescent and preadolescent sex play, those that enjoin girls to be modest, retiring, and submissive appear to produce adult women that are incapable or at least unwilling to be sexually aggressive . . . quite often they do not experience clear-cut sexual orgasm. In contrast, the societies which permit or encourage early sex play usually allow females a greater degree of freedom in seeking sexual contacts."[9] They found that these women when mature are generally more vigorous and aggressive during sex, which results in regular and satisfactory orgasms.[10]

Some cultures perform various puberty rites celebrating the development of adult sexuality. The erotic dances that frequently accompany these rites teach the art of lovemaking in pantomime. Our culture celebrates no comparable rites. However, our children can receive positive messages about sex from the obvious pleasure evidenced by their parents in the affectionate, playful, and loving gestures they extend to one another.

Another major concern of females, from childhood through adulthood, is physical beauty. For girls, being pretty, rather than plain, is considered all-important. Peers respond less critically and adults more favorably when you are pretty. As we approached adolescence, our feelings about our physical selves became particularly acute as we watched our bodies "develop" with each passing day. We would agonize and wonder how it would all end up. Would we have large or small breasts? What size would our waist or hips be? Would we always be taller than the boys? And we would constantly compare ourselves to our friends in an attempt to figure it out. While we were developing, it was almost as if our bodies were sabotaging us. We'd suddenly find a breast getting in the way where one had not interfered before. New pimples would develop despite the medications that guaranteed relief or your money back. We felt clumsy and awkward, far from the graceful high school girls we secretly emulated. There was no security in this new body that was becoming so different from the old comfortable one. We never knew what to expect next, as we asked the eternal question, would we be pretty?

Being attractive was of tremendous importance because it signaled love and acceptance, but it also presented a number of problems. While we longed to be attractive to the opposite sex, we had a lot of ambivalence about actually attracting them. Is it really OK to lure boys or are we bad and promiscuous if we do? The message was always mixed—yes and no. Our parents would respond with pride when we got all dressed up to visit relatives, but with suspicion if we were going out with our friends. The lipstick and eye makeup advertisements promised us popularity, but our wanting to use those products precipitated incessant battles at home. Finally after months or years of fighting, we may have won the right to cover our natural beauty in an attempt to be more attractive.

Many of us found ourselves overweight and constantly breaking the diets we had designed. Being overweight had its compensations; those of us who were fat did not have to compete in the sexual arenas where stakes were high. We could blame our weight for our lack of boyfriends and could nourish fantasies of how alluring we would be if only we lost the proper number of pounds. But we never put our fantasies to the test by slimming down; possibly we felt safer within the extra inches of armor. At least, we rationalized, we knew that the friends who liked us really liked us for ourselves, for our personalities, and not because of such superficial attributes as looks. While the thoughts that plagued pretty girls included: am I liked for myself, or just for my appearance?

Thus, appearance and appeal seemed to present a myriad of problems. If we were attractive, we may have worried about alienating other girls who were jealous of our looks, remembering well the lessons learned earlier that success at competition was not a favorable attribute for a girl. If we attracted boys we had the outside affirmation that we were, indeed, desirable, but we also became embarrassed over the attention and felt unsure about handling our admirers. If boys pursued us, we faced the dilemma of "putting out" or being labeled a tease or a prude. If he had an erection, we often felt we had to do something about it because we caused it. Walking the thin line between popularity and promiscuity wasn't easy.

We were led to believe that our sexual feelings for our boyfriends were wrong and bad. Boys were rightfully supposed to like sexual activities, while girls were not. How disconcerting it was to find out that many of us did when we weren't supposed to. So, many of us dutifully learned to keep our sexual feelings well under control or to suppress them altogether. When we were allowed to "date," it was clear that the responsibility for keeping things in line was ours. Boys were expected to "get away" with anything they could while we were supposed to stop them. Their sexuality was sanctioned; but a "good" girl was above sexuality, a cool creature of sensibility who knew how to control not only her own sexual feelings but her partner's as well, so she would not be "taken advantage of." We were taught that only "loose" girls participated in sex and that, while a boy could use these girls for his pleasure, he would never respect or marry a girl like that. A girl who acted on her sexual feelings would get a bad reputation while the boy would get a better one.

When I was a sixteen-year-old high school student, I attended a fraternity weekend with a boyfriend who was twenty-one and in college. We were at a New Jersey beach, and a beautiful day was coming to a close. As the evening grew longer and we grew more passionate, he earnestly implored me, "Never let me do anything to you that would make me lose respect for you." What a bind! Am I being too free in his eyes? Is this a warning about something he plans to try next? I was frightened and confused. Why couldn't he stop himself? Why did I have to figure out everything and keep the lid on tight?

Somehow, after years of practice at turning off sexual feelings both outwardly and inwardly, each of us is supposed to miraculously emerge as a turned-on, passionate woman when a legitimized adult sexual relationship materializes. Sally, one of the group members, realized that she desired sex more and felt more sexual sensations at sixteen than she did ten years later when she entered the group. She had learned to turn off her feelings very effectively while necking in the backseats of cars.

For many of us, the floodgates of our sexual feelings did not miraculously open when we finally started having intercourse. Even if our initiation into sex occurred on our wedding night, totally sanctioned by society and our parents, it may not have been easy to erase all the earlier negative messages that kept us anxious and overcontrolled.

Those of us who decided to go "all the way" before we were married may have had sex to prove our love to a boyfriend, or because we had run out of excuses and, exhausted by male pressure, found it easier to give in than continue to fight. Deciding to have sex because *he* wanted it was a fuzzy decision at best. Did we really want sex, too? Would he still respect us afterward? Or would he abandon us in the gutter as we were taught we deserved? And our worst fear was that he wouldn't keep it a secret, even though he had promised he would. We dreaded that he might even exaggerate his descriptions in locker room conversations, and that before we knew it, all our friends would know and our reputations would be forever ruined. All of these thoughts could produce enough anxiety and insecurity to prohibit relaxation and enjoyment of our first sexual experiences.

Even if we were strong enough to overcome the pressure of society and to decide on our own that making love was what we wanted for ourselves, the decision was often more easily accepted intellectually than emotionally. The 1972 Playboy Foundation Study indicates that more than half of the single females under 25 found their first coital experience as neutral or unpleasant. Only 20 percent said the first time was very pleasurable.[11]

Our first sexual experiences may have been good, bad, or indifferent. However, more than likely, we were self-conscious and embarrassed. Am I moving my body right? Am I making enough noise or am I too loud? Am I sexy? Would he rather be with so and so? And most of all, is he enjoying it and am I making it good for him? Not knowing what was in it for ourselves, we concentrated our energy on pleasing him and figuring out what he wanted us to do. Besides, we'd been much better trained at deciphering what someone else wanted and how to supply it than we were at making requests and obtaining pleasure for ourselves. So we ended up unsatisfied and wondered why there was so much fuss about sex anyway. At the other extreme, we may have experienced arousal to such an unaccustomed and intense degree the first time that it may have frightened us. As the rush of novel feelings threatened to overwhelm us, we may have frantically fought to maintain control.

Experiencing unsatisfying sex today is even more difficult than in the past because of the current demands on women to be sexually liberated. Societal pressure is making it harder and harder to say no, even if we don't feel we're ready for sex just yet. More and more younger women are sexually active according to a recent study. Approximately 46 percent of women experience intercourse before age eighteen and the trend, in general, is toward an earlier first intercourse.[12] But just because more women are sexually active these days doesn't mean that more are deriving adequate pleasure from sex.

Despite more liberal attitudes toward premarital sex, many women find themselves sexually experienced but not experiencing sex as comfortable and carefree. Janice used to laugh as required at a party when dirty jokes were being told; but the laughs were hollow and she secretly wished she knew what she was missing. To her, sex was just becoming a bigger and bigger drag.

An infinite number of events and experiences have contributed to your current sexual situation; each woman has been affected differently. Knowing how you got where you are may help you to realize that you're not the only one who feels as you do. "The Myth of the Vaginal Orgasm" by Ann Koedt, "The Politics of Orgasm" by Susan Lydon, and "Organs and Orgasm" by Alix Shulman are essays that may add additional perspective to the issues presented in these first two chapters.

3: Where Are You Now?

When we have to, we are all capable of finding ways of coping with a sexual situation that is unsatisfying. Many women have worked out compromises that enable them to endure sexual frustration, but these tend to be purely expedient measures which allow one to maintain a sex life at a bearable level, without actually solving the problem. Do you find yourself in this type of situation right now?

One common tendency is to get into the vicious cycle of expecting a sexual encounter to end with your feeling dissatisfied and frustrated, while hoping that *this* time it will be different. If so, you may find yourself being a spectator of your own lovemaking. As the lovemaking continues, you may grow more and more fearful that the orgasm is not going to happen. So you are constantly weighing your responses as you try to attain the elusive orgasm. The more closely you watch and worry, the less aware you can be of what your body is feeling. As your partner begins thrusting, you begin giving up. As he experiences orgasm, you may feel defeated, angry, sad, alone.

Ellen would find herself laughing uncontrollably after particularly frustrating episodes of lovemaking. Betty, on the other hand, would end up crying. But both women, after they had gone through these emotional stages, eventually felt almost nothing when lovemaking ended. They had learned to live without sexual enjoyment. It is unfortunate, though under-standable, that after consistent dissatisfaction with sex, if you can't see a solution to the problem, you begin to treat sex as a chore and attempt to avoid it or get it over with as quickly as possible.

You may find yourself sitting around patiently or impatiently waiting for "Mr. Right." You may be blaming your mother or father for not giving you the information you required or for instilling in you negative feelings about sex. You may be blaming your partner for not knowing enough or not caring enough. Or maybe you are beyond the point of caring whose fault it is, and like many women in the groups, have learned to "turn off" sexual feelings in an attempt to protect yourself from the inevitable frustration resulting from another incom-plete sexual experience. The earlier you turn off, the less frus-tration you may feel in the end. Some women learn to turn off so promptly that they experience no pleasurable sexual feelings at all.

Needless to say, under these conditions, the quicker sex is over, the better. You may have become an expert at making him come as quickly as possible. You know all the techniques that will excite your partner to orgasm, and you concentrate on these in order to get the lovemaking over. The faster he comes, the less time you are compelled to endure intercourse. But the more you focus on hurrying his orgasm, the less you concen-trate on your own experience. If you turn your sexual feelings off at the outset, there is no possibility you'll ever have an orgasm because you do not allow yourself to build on the small feelings you might experience if the process were to develop more slowly.

The most common method women use to cope with not reaching orgasm is to fake it. Many men will say that they don't believe a woman could successfully fake an orgasm, that they are certain they can tell the difference between a real orgasm and a faked orgasm. But can they really? Women have been faking orgasm successfully for years. But how can a woman learn how to fake an orgasm if she has never experienced a genuine one? Toni Ayres, one of my coworkers, learned by reading pornographic novels. The heroine would breathe hard, make deep gurgling sounds in her throat, and writhe about. So that was what she used to do. Carmen faked so successfully for two years that her partner never knew she wasn't orgasmic. She must have faked very convincingly, because even after she became orgasmic, she swore he couldn't tell the difference. He only noticed that she seemed to be enjoying sex more than ever.

Why do women fake orgasm? The reasons vary. Carmen and other women faked orgasm so that a partner wouldn't think they were inadequate. Do you fake because you're embarrassed and ashamed that you never have orgasms, or don't with any frequency, and you may not want anyone, especially your lover, to know. Maybe you're afraid he'll reject you. You may want his approval and think that responding to him sexually is one way to gain it. Another reason many women fake orgasm is to protect a partner's ego. Ellen's partner would try so hard to bring her to orgasm, she just didn't have the heart to let him down. You may somehow feel it's your duty to validate a partner's masculinity by showing him that he can satisfy you sexually. If you don't, you may fear he'll feel inadequate, be depressed, possibly even leave you. Still other women fake orgasm just to get the man to stop. If you know that a considerate male partner is trying to last until you achieve orgasm, and you know you aren't getting any closer, you may fake it— so that you can get him to stop thrusting and leave you alone.

But what price do you pay for faking orgasm? First, you

may be so busy faking that you end up totally missing the sexual feelings that you might otherwise perceive. After one group series was over, Janice said, "You know, I was faking so much, that it's possible that I had an orgasm, a little one, and didn't even know it." A second difficulty is that faking prevents your partner from learning that a problem exists. Unless you let him know that something is amiss, he will assume that his lovemaking techniques satisfy you. Consequently, he will continue doing the very things that have not been working. If you could let him know the truth, he might be willing to join you in trying out techniques that would prove more satisfying.

Finally, faking can be a trap because once you begin, it's hard to stop. The fear is that if you tell your partner he'll explode into rage or dissolve in hurt. Possibly you worry that he may feel he can't trust you again. But while there is a risk in admitting you've been faking, it's probably not so great as you might expect. If you explain yourself in a straightforward way, but without blaming him, chances are good that he'll respond with kindness and concern. However, if you tell him in anger, in the midst of a fight, you can expect the worst.

Sarah finally gained the courage to tell the man she had been living with for a year that she had never had an orgasm during that whole time. This couple had a particularly active sexual life. They frequently made love twice each day, and each time he would have two or three orgasms. He felt that he had to perform this way in order to satisfy her. When she told him that the thrusting of his penis was not the most sexually exciting thing for her, he was incredibly relieved. He then admitted that he had been faking some of those second and third orgasms because he thought that his coming inside her was what really turned her on. Thus, a double fake was in process. Both were trying to live up to what they assumed the other's expectations were, and consequently did not enjoy sex

body is able to participate sexually even if she's not sexually aroused. For men, the penis can say no. Nevertheless many men, and an even greater number of women, endure the emotional and physical discomforts of making love at times when they're not really interested.

Of course, it is possible to find some payoff in using unsatisfactory sex as a way of punishing your partner. You don't have an orgasm and he feels sorry, or by grudgingly going along with sex in a passive and disinterested way, you keep him from enjoying sex as much as he might if you, too, were really involved.

Where does all this leave you? Even though the media, the women's movement, and contraceptive availability have changed some attitudes, you may still feel inadequate and insecure about trying anything new. Perhaps you don't want to broadcast your "deficiency." Or, you may be left sacrificing your own pleasure in order to please a partner, protecting his ego so he won't feel inadequate. It almost surely leaves you demoralized, without a solution to the problem. Maybe you're convinced you will never enjoy sex fully or reach orgasm.

If you are caught in any of these binds, there are solutions, and we'll explore them in the chapters to follow. Since sex is just a basic form of communication and lack of sexual communication may be indicative of other communication failures in your relationship, it may be best to begin by discussing the problem with your partner, just as soon as you feel ready to, so that your partner understands what's going on and can join you in seeking a solution. But most of all you need to decide to *do something about it yourself*, beyond complaining and waiting for your partner to take action, or waiting for some miracle to occur. Trying something new is the first big step. For example, is intercourse really the only way to make love? What are some of the things you might suggest to a partner that might help?

Some of the exercises in Chapters 8, 9, 12, and 13 are one approach, but it's up to you to do the talking, to take the initiative. By understanding where you are now, and seeing how your particular ways of coping with sexual frustration actually prevent you from solving the problem, you may find the courage to experiment and change your sexual life. Masters and Johnson have helped redefine sexuality by describing the actual process of the sexual response cycle in women. Each woman needs to build on that basic information (contained in Chapter 5) and discover her unique sexual pattern, and then share this knowledge with her lover.

4: The First Steps Toward Change

I talked with a colleague, Leah Potts, about the many negative sex messages and experiences women have to overcome in order to become more sexually responsive. "You know," she said, "the whole thing just wouldn't seem worth the effort—except that it feels *sooo* good."

One way to get beyond the negative sex attitudes you may have developed is by finding out what they are and, if possible, where they come from. Certainly, you may not be able to unravel all the tangled strands; some of the messages may have been so indirect they remain only vague feelings that you are unable to trace back to anything specific.

But nevertheless, there are a number of ways to go about reexploring your sexual past. One good way is to sit down with a close female friend and describe to one another sexual attitudes and experiences you had while you were growing up. The women in the groups found this exercise especially helpful. By talking with another woman, as opposed to a man, it is easier to reach a deeper level of understanding because of the common history of growing up female. Although a man might be able to appreciate and understand you, his understanding would not be based on his personal experience. Nonetheless, there are some advantages to discussing your sexual history with a good male friend, or lover, too. Doing so can make the relationship closer and more intimate; it can deepen the level of trust between the two of you; it can give you further understanding of what has gone into shaping the personality of the person with whom you are so close. Opening up communication through a detailed discussion of your sexual history can provide a good starting point for the two of you to begin talking about sex more openly with each other and for understanding one another's needs. If there is no one with whom you feel comfortable discussing these issues, try writing down your thoughts. Or, at least set aside some time alone in which to explore your thoughts in depth.

The following topics should provide a good starting point for exploring your attitudes and development as a sexual being: 1) How did your parents feel about sex? Your mother? Your father? How were their feelings communicated to you? 2) What was the attitude of your peers toward sex as you were growing up? 3) When and how did you learn about menstruation? What was the attitude of the person who told you? Were you frequently very uncomfortable—cramps? Were you ever embarrassed by an incident involving menstruation? 4) When and how did you learn about masturbation? Do you remember when you first masturbated? 5) When and how did you learn what sex really was? Were you shocked? 6) What were the circumstances of your first real sexual experience and what was it like for you? 7) Any sexual traumas such as child-adult sexual contact, rape, or other frightening sexual experiences? Spend five to ten minutes on each question. (For additional exercises of this nature, refer to Roberta and Herbert Otto's book, *Total Sex*.)

Some colleagues found that another area of exploration which proved to be very important to the women in the groups was a direct discussion with their mothers about sex. Telephone your mother or visit her if either is possible. Begin the discussion by asking her what *her* mother (your grandmother) told her about sex and contraception when she got married. This information can be productive for a number of reasons. First, it can help to put your mother's personal attitudes toward sex in perspective—especially if they have been negative. Second, you may learn some things about your mother and her sexuality that may differ from your expectations, and this may enable you to reevaluate your impressions. Third, this discussion can grow in breadth and depth to include early experiences, conversations, events—things you may have forgotten about or things you always wanted to share but never had the opportunity or courage to initiate. Most important, it can give you a real framework, negative or positive, in which to view your sexual development. This aspect of placing fantasies in perspective can be a very positive learning experience.

In *The Sensuous Woman*, "J" wrote: "Pin up on your bed, your mirror, your wall, a sign, lady, until you know it in every part of your being: We are designed to delight, excite, and satisfy the male of the species."[1] I would like to add that we were designed to be delighted, excited, and satisfied ourselves. Nina always had a smile on her face and never voiced any dissatisfaction to her husband. She always tried to make the best of things and totally withheld anger and disappointment. She feared that if she expressed any negative feelings, he would stop loving her. She was so practiced at withholding her feelings that her sexual feelings didn't get expressed either and she never experienced an orgasm. It was amazing to her that when she began to express her dissatisfaction with other areas of the relationship, she began having orgasms as well.

You deserve pleasure, but pleasure may be difficult to allow yourself to take. You may feel you don't deserve it or that other things are more pressing or important, so you leave yourself out.

Developing your sexual potential means finding time to

devote to sex; for most women this means allotting the time from busy schedules. But to make the time and accept pleasure, you have to feel you deserve it, that you are important, too, as important as those you love and care for. It's necessary to give to yourself as well as to others. If you always have to be the good, strong, giving one, you can't help being angry at times about getting the short end of the deal. Sarah had been well trained to wait on men and she was good at it. She was a good seamstress, a good cook, and a caring and selfless companion. But she ended up resenting her partner and the fact that he thought he could repay her by making love to her. Without even realizing it, she found herself thinking, "You think you're so hot, I'll show you. I won't have an orgasm." Surely there are benefits to being a selfless, martyred servant. Because you wait on him, he is indebted to you. Perhaps you'll be worth so much to him that he'll never risk leaving you. But you end up cheating yourself. It's unlikely that he stays with you just because you're a good servant. Ellen was angry at her husband but kept being the good "wifey," as she put it. In the group Lydia told Ellen, "You've got a right to live. You're not serving time. Be good to yourself. Be kind to yourself. You deserve it. It's a matter of survival." Lydia added that she had always thought it was better to give than to receive. "I used to give things away to be liked. You know, that's a bunch of horseshit. I deserve something for myself, too."

You have a right to refuse things you don't want and ask for things you do want. You may feel you deserve and want more for yourself, but don't know how to go about having your needs met. Here is an exercise that has been beneficial to virtually every woman with whom I've worked.

The exercise is called yes's and no's. Doing the no's entails saying no to three things you didn't want to do anyway, but would usually agree to do. It could mean saying no to someone who has asked you to do something that you don't really want to do. For example, Ann said no to a woman from a charity who wanted Ann to go out collecting money for them. Ann always hated doing it, but had never refused before. This time she did and felt relieved. This exercise can also include saying no to yourself. In other words, you can refuse to do something you feel you *should* do but don't want to do. For example, Laura always cleaned her house on Saturdays, but on this particular Saturday, she was exhausted from a busy week and just didn't feel like doing it. She really felt like going out shopping instead, so she said no to the "I should clean house" and enjoyed her day.

Try saying no to at least three things in the next few days. You can say no to yourself or to someone else, but it's important to do at least one of each. Sarah always felt she had to go to bed with the men she was steadily dating, even if she didn't want to on a particular night. She was afraid if she refused that she would lose them. She decided to take a risk and began telling her lovers, before she even went out for the evening, that she did not want to have sex for a while and that she would tell them when she felt like it. To her amazement her request was honored and respected. One lover did try to push her to make love, but she held firm and not one man ended the relationship because of her refusal to have sex for the period of time she needed to feel that she was back in control of her life.

The yes's are just the opposite of the no's. Doing the yes's entails saying yes to three things that you really want but would not normally let yourself have or would not usually allow yourself to ask others for. Eve splurged and bought herself a sweater she had been admiring, but felt was too expensive to buy for herself. Barbara asked her husband to make dinner one night when she was tired. She had never considered asking him to do something like that before. Joy was going to be thirty-five in a week and felt this was a very important point in her life. She asked some of her friends if they would make something special for her, for this birthday, and ended up receiving some beautiful handcrafted gifts.

Experiment with the yes's and no's and see how you feel after doing them. Remember, you should select things you would not normally refuse or request. If you would have said yes or no anyway, it doesn't count; the point of the exercise is to help you do some things differently, to be more self-assertive. Some women can perform the no's easily but have difficulty with the yes's. For other women the problem is just the reverse, and many women have trouble with both. Practice the one(s) you have difficulty with a few times more. Don't berate yourself or become discouraged when you realize that you let an opportunity go by. Missing opportunities is a good way to see just how often you fail to permit yourself the freedom to do or not do what you want. You may see how much of yourself you deny for others. Louise thought that doing the yes's and no's would be easy for her. She felt further ahead of the other women in the group. Then she realized she had a stomachache. She said, "If I let myself, I'm going to get in touch with all the things that are similar to the other women and it's going to be hard and may take a while." Each woman must begin where she is and go at her own pace. Only you know how far and how fast you can push yourself without considerable discomfort.

Feeling you deserve more for yourself is necessary in order to develop your sexuality. If you don't feel you deserve the pleasure, you won't set aside the time necessary to attain it. If you don't set aside the time to practice, nothing will change.

In addition to revisiting your sexual past, and feeling you deserve more for yourself, it is imperative that you get back in touch with your body. Any alienation you may experience in this regard can be as much the result of socialization, which taught you to keep your body discreetly covered, as the media messages that dictate how you should look. (We are bombarded with ads that ask: Are you clean and hairless? Do you smell just right in all the proper places, or should you buy such and such a product to enhance your appeal?) Have you ever stopped to think just whom you are grooming yourself for? Is it for you, for him, or for the advertising agencies?

You may be alienated from the sight of your body. When was the last time you really looked closely at your body? Many of us avoid looking because we see only the imperfections— imperfections which magazines, television, movies, etc. have taught us to recognize. Mass media, and designers of women's clothing, set different standards for what a woman should look like each year. If we are not this year's model, we are made to feel dissatisfied with ourselves. We accept the blatant fallacy that unless we look like a twenty-year-old Playboy bunny, we're not sexually attractive. Wide hips were "in" one decade and large breasts the next. Now, we're all expected to be flat-chested beanpoles. If your body type is "in" one year, it's "out" the next. To try to rearrange your body to fit the times is, of course, absurd. Furthermore, few people applaud the natural body changes that accompany the processes of aging and childbearing. It's time to stop thinking that the problem lies within ourselves and start wondering why the media is trying to cut all of us out with the same cookie cutter rather than encouraging us to capitalize on our uniqueness.

Very few of us have the current "ideal figure," and there is no reason why we should even attempt to conform. It's important to get to know your own body, to become friends with it even if there are a few improvements you would like to make. The women in the groups found the process of reexperiencing their bodies in a new and different way an invaluable one.

How can you get back in touch with your body? One good exercise is to set up a full-length mirror in the privacy of your room. Lock your door and undress in front of it. Carefully examine your body. You might talk to yourself while you're looking, telling yourself what you see. Look at your body from all angles, standing, kneeling, sitting with legs apart and together. Look at yourself for a minimum of fifteen minutes. Seeing what your lover sees when he looks at you might make you less embarrassed and inhibited. Some women are preoccupied with making sure the lights are out and that their bodies are safely hidden under the covers before they can relax and get into a sexual mood.

When a partner does caress your body do you remain concerned about whether he likes it or not? Do you have a tendency to rearrange yourself to keep what you consider your worst attributes concealed? Playing the artful dodger is certainly not conducive to a relaxed, open, and enjoyable sexual encounter.

If you believe your partner has negative feelings about your body or is not quite comfortable with it, you might try asking him about it and discussing it together. You may learn that you're far more critical of yourself than others are of you or you may learn that you have realistically appraised the situation. You may or may not want to change certain aspects of your body. In any case, talking about it together can help keep things in perspective.

Many women in the groups had difficulty carrying out the mirror exercise at first. Expecting the worst, they procrastinated to avoid confronting their fears. However, few women found the actual exercise to be as disconcerting as they had expected. Most women have not looked at their bodies long enough to examine their negative feelings about the image reflected in the mirror. Cindy did not want to do the mirror exercise because she was a bit overweight. We pointed out that just because she avoided looking didn't mean the weight would not be there. It was important for her to know the body she walked around in each day, even if it was changing. Eventually she carefully studied her body, and to her surprise, she found that she actually liked it, despite the extra weight. Cindy rarely goes on diets anymore. The few extra pounds don't seem to matter now that her attitude about her body has changed and she has learned to accept it. Some women find that looking at their own bodies really turns them on. Get to know your body so you feel free to enjoy it more fully.

After you've examined yourself carefully in the mirror for at least fifteen minutes, begin to explore your body with your hands. Again, try talking to yourself, this time about what your hands are feeling. Ms. Jeremy Brav made this suggestion to the women in one of her groups: "Pretend you're from another planet landing on this unknown body for the first time. Your assignment is to explore this new body completely." Run your fingers over your arms, legs, stomach, etc.; feel the muscles, the bones, the fat, and the varied textures of skin. Compare the skin on your inner thigh to that on the soles of your feet, to that on your lips, ears, chest, shins, buttocks. Enjoy the feelings of your hands touching your skin as well as your skin being touched. See if you can't discover something you didn't know before. Do you like any areas of your body better than you thought you would? Can you begin to accept the fact that it's OK to look the way you do? Leslie told the group, "I feel a whole lot better about my body. We're not quite *good* friends yet, but we're friends."

Understanding and accepting the way you are now—your mind and how it has developed through upbringing and experience, your body and how you look and feel physically—are the first steps toward understanding and accepting yourself as a person with a unique sexual nature.

5: The Anatomy and Physiology of Female Sexuality

In order to understand how a woman functions sexually, it is important to distinguish between the various parts of the female genitals, and to see how each part works. The following is a very brief description of female sexual anatomy to help you locate the various structures; the diagram on the next page can be used as a guide.

The most external structure of the female genitals, the fleshy outer lips (labia majora) are covered with pubic hair. Within these outer lips are the inner lips which cover the vaginal and urethral openings when the woman is not sexually excited. At the point at which the inner lips are joined together at the top, there is a small pink structure, varying in size, but often about the size of a tiny pea. This structure is called the glans of the clitoris, and it is a very important structure in female sexuality.

It may be difficult to find the clitoris at first because it is covered by a hood called the prepuce. The clitoral shaft extends beneath the hood to the glans of the clitoris. Below the clitoris and above the vaginal opening is the urethra. This small hole, through which urine is expelled, is also sometimes difficult to locate. The easiest way to find it is to put your finger inside your vagina and pull the opening down toward the anus. The

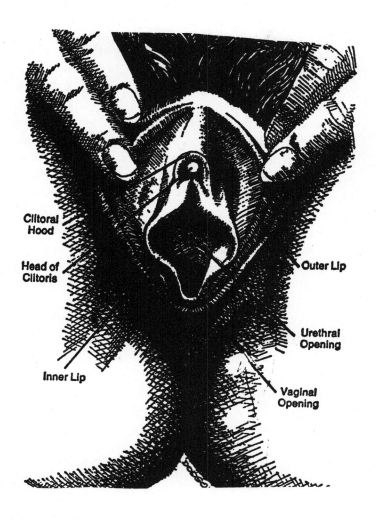

Clitoral
Hood

Head of
Clitoris

Inner Lip

Outer Lip

Urethral
Opening

Vaginal
Opening

urethra will generally appear from within the folds of skin. Below the urethra is the vaginal opening. The area between the vagina and the anus is called the perineum.

The illustration on page 49 shows one woman's genitals. Each woman's genitals are unique. That is, while women have the same basic structures, these structures vary considerably, from woman to woman, in size, color, shape; and the structures vary in distance from one another. The genitals have a configuration as unique as our faces: we all have eyes, a nose, and a mouth, but they vary in size and placement. Some of us have large noses, but this doesn't mean we can smell better; small eyes don't imply inferior vision. These differences, however, do play a part in making each of us unique in appearance. The same is true of the genitals. The "faces" of our genitals are distinct. However, the size or the placement of the different structures does not seem to have much effect on sexual functioning.[1] Some women have large puffy outer lips while others have very thin outer lips. In some women the outer lips take on a hue that is just slightly darker than the area around it. Some women have a lot of pubic hair and others have little, and the color of a woman's pubic hair can differ in color from the hair on her head (just as the color of the hair in a man's beard often differs from the color of the hair on his head).

The size of the clitoris also varies somewhat among women. In some African tribes little girls elongate the clitoris either through pulling or some other artificial method because a large clitoris is supposed to be a sign of beauty. Some women have a small bump on the glans of their clitoris; or their clitoris is split, resulting in two separate but attached pieces. The hood over the clitoris can vary considerably in size and fleshiness. The clitoral hood of some women has many folds while others are very simple and small. The inner lips vary as well. Some women have very narrow inner lips, while others have long inner lips that hang below the outer lips. The inner lips vary in color from pink to brown; and some women even have two-toned inner lips—pink on the inner part with brown toward the edges. None of these variations seems to affect the ability of a woman to respond sexually.

One of my favorite stories is one I heard from an artist friend. As a young girl she examined her genitals and found that one of her inner lips was longer than the other. She assumed that this must have been caused by masturbation. Rather than stopping masturbating, she decided to concentrate the stimulation on the side that had the smaller inner lip and, in this way, attempt to even them out. As you might guess, she never did succeed in evening out the lips. The discrepancy wasn't caused by masturbation, but was one of the unique features of her genitals.

Now that the various areas of your genitals have been designated, it is important to understand the ways in which these different structures function sexually.

For most women the urethra is one of the least important structures from the point of view of sexual stimulation. Stimulation of the area just outside the urethra can be enjoyable and sexually arousing for some women, while others just find it irritating. The urethra usually goes unnoticed in most women until some bladder infection or infection of the urethra develops, causing misery. It may itch, burn, or irritate in a way that makes the woman feel that she needs to urinate, even when she doesn't have to. Infections of this type and other gynecological disorders can often be prevented by a few simple health techniques. After you go to the bathroom, wipe the anal and vaginal areas separately to prevent bacteria in one area from infecting the other. Drink water before intercourse and urinate before and after having intercourse. This cleans out the urethra and helps to prevent infections from occurring.

The vagina is just below the urethra. The closeness of these two structures may account for some of the confusing messages girls received while growing up. Since most of us didn't know there were two openings down there, we associated the entire genital area with urination. Urinating was something private, and we were apologetic when we excused ourselves to go to the bathroom. So it is possible that at some level we ended up confusing our sexual and excretory functions.

The sexual sensitivity of the vagina varies with the individual woman. However, nerve endings that respond to touch are only contained near the entrance.[2] Therefore, the walls of the first third of the vagina are more responsive to sexual stimulation than those of the inner two thirds. The inner two thirds is sensitive to stretch and pressure,[3] and many women get considerable pleasure from this area during the deep thrusting that takes place during intercourse. Since it is the outer third of the vagina that is most sensitive, however, almost any penis is large enough to stimulate this area. Even though the size of an erect penis, regardless of its size when flaccid, varies very little from man to man,[4] it is true that some women have a preference for a larger or a smaller penis. However, a large penis does not necessarily make a man a better lover.

This idea of preference in sexual matters is a very important one. We accept the idea that different people prefer certain foods; preferences for specific foods reflect individual differences of constitution, temperament, or past experience. The same holds true for preferences in sexual stimulation. There are differences in the actual quality and types of nerve endings existing in the various areas of each woman's genitals;[5] these anatomical differences may account, in part, for the difference in sexual preferences.

Preferences can also be learned; they can result from the experiences of touching yourself, information, and misinformation resulting from things you've read or from what friends have said. You may be capable of having orgasms in a number of positions, but prefer, for whatever reason, a particular position. Your task is to discern or begin to learn about your unique preferences in sexual stimulation, as you do every day in food or dress.

Another important physical characteristic of the vagina is the large muscle that surrounds the opening and covers the whole pelvic floor (from the pubic bone to the tail bone). It is called the pubococcygeal muscle, or "PC muscle," and it is one of the muscles that contracts during orgasm. If you put your finger into the entrance to your vagina and/or the entrance to your anus during an orgasm, you usually can feel the rhythmic contractions of this muscle. The PC muscle may be lacking in tone in some women, especially after childbirth. Like any other muscle, the PC muscle needs exercise to keep it in its best condition. A series of exercises popularly referred to as "Kegels" were developed by Dr. Arnold Kegel for women with the common problem of urinary incontinence.[6] These women would expel urine when they sneezed or coughed and the Kegel exercises were designed to tighten the PC muscle, and help them contain the urine. Many gynecologists recommend Kegels routinely to women after they have had a baby.[7] "Kegeling" is also taught in many natural childbirth classes.

Some of the women who followed Dr. Kegel's advice reported that after about six weeks of practicing the exercises they experienced increased pleasure during sexual intercourse. The women I have worked with have also found that exercising the PC muscle increases sensitivity in the vaginal area. In addition, strengthening this muscle helps reduce spontaneous urination with orgasm, an occurrence which is not unusual among women. I highly recommend that you practice the following Kegel exercises.

To locate your pubococcygeal muscle, urinate with your legs apart; the muscle you squeeze to stop the flow of urine is the PC muscle. Practice stopping the flow of urine a few times in order to become familiar with the muscle. Then lie down and put your finger in the opening of your vagina and contract the PC muscle. See if you can feel the contraction around your finger.

After practicing the following exercises for about six weeks, see if you notice any difference in the strength of your PC muscle when you put your finger in your vagina and squeeze.

The first Kegel exercise consists of squeezing the PC muscle for three seconds, then relaxing the muscle for three seconds, and squeezing it again. Begin with ten three-second squeezes at three different times during the day. It may be difficult at first to keep contracting for a full three seconds. If that is the case, contract for one or two seconds and build up the time as the muscle gets stronger.

The advantage to these exercises is that you can do them anywhere and at any time and no one can tell you're doing them. Practice when you stop the car for a red light or in the morning when you wake up. Or do them when you answer the telephone at home or at work, or when you are lying down to rest. The muscles surrounding your anus may also contract during the exercise, but if you find that you are moving your thigh muscles, your stomach or buttocks, you are probably squeezing the wrong muscle.

The second exercise is like the first except that the objective is to squeeze the muscle, release it, squeeze again and release as quickly as possible. This is nicknamed the "flutter" exercise. Again, squeeze and release ten times at three different times during the day. When you first start doing this exercise, it may feel like a tongue twister; you may not be able to tell if you are contracting or releasing and for a while it may keep getting muddled all together. However, after working at it slowly, you will gradually be able to do the flutter more rapidly.

The third exercise consists of imagining that there is a tampon at the opening to the vagina and that you are sucking it up into your vagina. Gloria was actually able to suck water into her vagina and then spurt it out again when she did this exercise while taking a bath.

The fourth exercise consists of bearing down as during a bowel movement, but with the emphasis more on the vagina than the anal area. This exercise is more apparent to an observer. Both the sucking in and the bearing down should be held for three seconds, as with the first exercise.

All four exercises should be practiced ten times each at three different times during the day. Attend equally to relaxing and contracting the muscle. As you progress with these Kegel exercises, slowly increase the number in each series until you are able to do twenty of each exercise in succession. You can do them as frequently during the day as you can find time, but consider three times daily a minimum.

If you notice some discomfort or tightness in the pelvic area at the beginning, reduce the number of daily contractions, but do not abandon the exercises. Like any muscle that is being exercised for the first time, it may get a little stiff at first. It is quite important to keep this muscle, like others in your body, in tone. The exercises can become as much of a habit as brushing your teeth and, like brushing your teeth, they should be continued for the rest of your life.

The anus is also a very sensitive area for some, but not all women. Some women enjoy having this area lightly stroked or licked during lovemaking. Some women enjoy the insertion of a finger in the anus while having intercourse and others enjoy having their partner's penis inserted into the anus instead of the vagina.

But for many, if not most, women, the most important site of sexual sensitivity is the clitoral area. Recent research indicates that two thirds of the women studied preferred and responded more readily to clitoral than vaginal stimulation.[8] The fact that the clitoris is usually more sensitive to sexual stimulation than the vagina is because the density of nerve endings in the clitoris is far greater than it is in the vagina. Kelly was relieved to learn this fact. She said that it was good to know that it wasn't her fault that she had been feeling very little sexual excitement during intercourse.

The entire area above, to the sides, and below the clitoris is generally highly sensitive to sexual stimulation. However, the exact areas that provide the most pleasure differ from woman to woman. Embryologically, the glans of the penis and glans of the clitoris developed from the same tissue.[9] Therefore, because it is small, the glans of the clitoris actually has a higher density of nerve endings than the glans (or head) of the male penis.

The clitoris has no other function than that of providing the woman with sexual pleasure.[10] Laurie, a very religious woman, had some initial difficulty accepting the fact that it was the clitoris and not the vagina that was the primary seat of sexual excitement in most women. She explored the area with her fingers and found it to be true for her. Since the clitoris has no function other than providing sexual pleasure, she reasoned that God must have meant it to be there so that the woman would enjoy sex. Otherwise God wouldn't have put it there. Laurie's explanation seems to persuade other religious women with whom I have subsequently worked that sexual pleasure and religious morality are compatible.

The inner lips are attached to the prepuce or hood covering the clitoris and to the clitoris itself. During intercourse, the thrusting of the penis in and out of the vagina pulls on the inner lips which in turn pull on the hood of the clitoris. This movement of the hood back and forth over the sensitive clitoris provides sexual pleasure for most women during intercourse. Check this for yourself by tugging on the inner lips and by inserting several fingers in and out of the vagina. Since both the vaginal and clitoral areas are being stimulated simultaneously during intercourse, it is often difficult for women to discern exactly where the pleasurable stimulation is coming from. Once the importance of the clitoris is understood, it is easy to see why the indirect stimulation of this area provided by intercourse is frequently insufficient to enable a woman to reach orgasm.

The clitoral area may also receive stimulation from the rubbing of the male's pelvic bone against the clitoris during intercourse, but again, this nonspecific stimulation may be insufficient to enable a woman to have an orgasm through thrusting alone.

In order to reach orgasm, many, if not most, women require additional direct stimulation of either the glans or the shaft of the clitoris or the adjacent areas. It makes no more sense to justify the necessity of direct stimulation of the female sex organ, the clitoris, than it does to justify the need for direct stimulation of the male sex organ, the penis, in order for an orgasm to occur. Somehow, we have accepted the myth that additional clitoral stimulation, beyond that provided in intercourse, should be unnecessary or is unnatural. The belief is that the penis should produce the orgasm; but if the penis does not produce enough direct pressure to stimulate the woman's most sensitive area, it seems sensible to add stimulation that does.

Some women find it difficult to slide the hood back and forth easily over the clitoris. This can be caused by the gathering of natural secretions called smegma, which can get trapped under the clitoral hood where they may dry and harden if the area is not washed regularly. These crystals of smegma can make clitoral stimulation painful. The effect is similar to rubbing your eyelid when sand is caught underneath. Smegma can be removed by washing the area. In a small minority of women, tiny membranes called clitoral adhesions can attach the clitoris to the hood, preventing the hood from moving freely back and forth across the clitoris. By using a dull probe, a doctor can sever these attaching membranes in a simple office procedure. It has not been satisfactorily established, however, whether this minor operation plays an important part in enabling a woman to experience orgasm.[11] Some women do report having been helped by this procedure; and yet, many women with clitoral adhesions report no difficulty whatsoever reaching orgasm. Again, women respond differently.

While clitoral stimulation is generally required to attain orgasm, there are exceptions. About 2 percent of the female population, according to Kinsey, are capable of having an orgasm through fantasy alone, with no accompanying genital stimulation; another small percentage can experience orgasm through breast or other nongenital stimulation.[12] Some women have experienced spontaneous orgasms and many women have had orgasms while dreaming. However, despite these exceptions, a substantial amount of stimulation of the genital area is the necessary prelude to orgasm for the majority of women. The exact area and type of genital stimulation needed for orgasm depends upon the physiological makeup and learned response patterns of each individual woman. Let's assume that two women have comparable emotional involvement with a man. His lovemaking technique might arouse the first woman, but exactly the same approach and type of stimulation might do nothing for the second.

Again, we are talking about preference. Some women prefer direct and hard stimulation of the glans of the clitoris or the surrounding area, while others find this kind of stimulation irritating and enjoy a lighter touch. Preferences for timing and sequence, for setting and mood also vary from woman to woman. As my coworker Leah Potts puts it, "If you want to make beautiful music with me, you'll have to learn my song."

Physiologically, an orgasm is an orgasm, whether it occurs during masturbation, intercourse, oral stimulation, or any other form of stimulation. The subjective experience may differ, but the physiological cycle a woman goes through as she builds sexual tension, reaches orgasm, and returns to the initial resting place is the same for all women. This process, called the sexual response cycle, was detailed by Masters and Johnson as the result of the scientific observation of numerous women in their laboratory in St. Louis, Missouri.[13]

For purposes of description Masters and Johnson divided the sexual response cycle into four general phases: the excitement phase, the plateau phase, the orgasmic phase, and the resolution phase. We now know that a fifth phase, the desire phase, precedes these other four. These phases are not totally discrete. There is no distinct end to one phase before the next phase begins. Instead the phases represent an effort to describe a sequence of reactions that characteristically occur in what is really a continuous process.

Before sexual excitement commences, the female sexual organs are in what is called the resting state. The inner lips are flaccid, covering the vaginal opening; the vagina is more a potential space than an actual space. Like a balloon that has not yet been inflated, the walls of the vagina are relaxed and touching.

As the woman becomes sexually aroused through fantasy, emotions, contact with her lover, self-stimulation, or any other form of stimulation, the excitement phase begins. Blood starts to accumulate in the pelvic area just as blood accumulates to make our faces red when we blush.

In addition to the engorgement of the sexual organs with blood, a number of other processes occur during the excitement phase. The first is of vaginal lubrication. Through the use of a clear phallic-shaped camera which was inserted into the vagina during masturbation, Masters and Johnson learned that most of the lubricant was actually exuded by the walls of the vagina in a process similar to sweating. This lubrication process, a response to the rise in vaginal temperature produced by increased blood supply, is one of the first signs of sexual arousal in a woman, just as an erection is one of the first obvious signs of a male's arousal. Lubrication is generally present internally before it reaches the vaginal orifice. Anxiety, contraceptive pills, certain drugs—including antihistamines and decongestants—and hormonal changes are some of the influences that can inhibit lubrication even when a woman feels turned on. In these cases saliva, K-Y Jelly, and Astroglide, or some other lubricant can be used. The presence of lubrication does not necessarily indicate that the woman is sufficiently aroused to want intercourse to begin, although many men interpret the presence of lubrication as a signal for penile insertion. And the presence of lubrication is certainly no indication that a woman is close to having an orgasm. She might be able to have intercourse at this point without it being unpleasant, but it would probably be much more pleasurable if she waited and continued other forms of stimulation first.

As sexual stimulation continues, the vagina expands and lengthens. The elastic capacity of the walls of the vagina are impressive. The vaginal space can compress enough for the walls to hold a tampon snugly and expand sufficiently to permit the birth of a baby. As the vaginal canal expands, the uterus, which naturally extends into the back of the vagina, tips forward and up, providing enough space to accommodate a penis. The most common cause of the discomfort that can sometimes occur during deep thrusting is the impact of the penis against the mouth of the cervix. The cervical mouth itself is not very sensitive, but contact with it can cause the attached uterus to move, and the resulting pressure on the ligaments that hold the uterus in place may cause the pain a woman sometimes feels. Switching coital positions can help eliminate discomfort.

The accumulation of blood in the pelvic area causes the tissues to swell in much the same way a sponge swells when it is filled with water. The outer lips, inner lips, clitoris, and sometimes the breasts, begin to look puffier and slightly enlarged in size. In some, but not all, women the nipples become erect. Late in the excitement phase, the darker skin surrounding the nipples, called the areolas, begin to swell also.

As the sexual excitement continues, the female experiences some changes that are characteristic of what Masters and Johnson call the plateau phase. The outer lips may become even puffier as she approaches orgasm. The tissues of the walls of the outer third of the vagina, including the PC muscle, swell with blood and a narrowing of the space at the vaginal opening results. The affected area is called the orgasmic platform. This constriction of the vaginal opening can intensify the pleasure of the male partner because his penis, when inserted, often feels as if it is being snugly held. At about this time, the clitoris may appear to be lost somewhere beneath the hood; you may wonder where it has gone and search for it in order to continue clitoral stimulation. However, the clitoris does continue to respond to direct stimulation of the area around it.

As arousal continues, breathing and pulse rates increase. A "sex flush" may become visible at some point during the plateau phase, but it doesn't appear on everyone. This flush is a measles-like rash that generally spreads over the stomach, breasts, shoulders, neck, or face area. The extent and description of the sex flush varies widely among women. The areolas surrounding the nipples may swell even further. Sometimes this area swells to such an extent that, in comparison, the nipples do not look erect. Many muscles—the facial muscles, thigh muscles, hand and foot muscles—may automatically and noticeably tense up. Many women consciously tense up even further the muscles in the pelvic area, the buttocks and thighs, to heighten their sexual pleasure.

The above descriptions generally accompany the plateau phase, but the extent to which each sign is visible depends upon the individual woman and to some extent the particular situation. The one definite and dependable sign of an imminent orgasm is a change in the color of the inner lips, not the easiest sign to discern during lovemaking. For women who have never had children, the inner lips turn from pink to bright red and, in women who have had children, from bright red to a deep purple or wine color.

After this change in color, if effective stimulation is continued, the woman will move into the orgasmic phase. Breathing, pulse rate, and blood pressure will continue to rise until a body reflex reverses the process of progressively increased muscle tension and blood supply to the sexual tissues. You cannot force an orgasm any more than you can force a knee jerk; both reflexes happen naturally. The mounting muscular tension and engorgement of blood vessels reaches a peak and orgasm occurs. The first third of the vaginal barrel, the PC muscle that has formed the orgasmic platform, contracts rhythmically approximately every 0.8 seconds for a brief period. The number and strength of the contractions vary in accordance with the intensity of the orgasm. The muscles of the uterus, and the anal sphincter muscle, may also contract more or less strongly.

These contractions may be apparent externally as the abdominal area appears to contract in waves or spasms. In many women, these contractions are barely, if at all, noticeable. The orgasm may be accompanied by a reflex grasping-type muscular response of the hands and feet. Some women may experience a feeling of warmth emanating from the genital area. The sensation of warmth results from the release of the blood from the engorged blood vessels of the pelvic region. The orgasm triggers the release of blood, allowing it to return to other areas of the body, and the resolution phase begins.

Regardless of what type of stimulation the woman receives, her body will progress through the physiological phases of the sexual response cycle. Whether the orgasm occurs through clitoral stimulation alone, through manual masturbation, through use of a vibrator, through lovemaking with another female, as the result of intercourse with a male partner, or fantasy alone, the reactions that comprise the cycle of excitement, plateau, orgasm, and resolution will proceed as described.

The Freudian distinction between the "vaginal" and "clitoral" orgasm does not match scientific findings. Every orgasm manifests itself in the whole pelvic region regardless of the part of the body that has been stimulated. If you have an orgasm once through intercourse alone with no accompanying direct clitoral stimulation and another time through oral sex, it would be erroneous to label the first a vaginal orgasm and the second a clitoral orgasm. Both are simply orgasms. Both involve the same set of responses. The subjective experience of the orgasm may vary according to the woman's mood, her feelings about her partner or about masturbation, the duration of stimulation, etc., but the physiological process of the buildup and release of sexual tension remains more or less the same. In the words of Masters and Johnson, "From an anatomic point of view, there is absolutely no difference in the responses of the pelvic viscera to effective sexual stimulation regardless of whether the stimulation occurs as a result of clitoral body or mons pubis area manipulation, natural or artificial coition, or, for that matter, specific stimulation of any other erogenous area of the female body."[14]

Since orgasm is usually triggered by genital, and more specifically clitoral, stimulation, the excitement usually stops if the stimulation stops. Stopping the stimulation does not cause the excitement level to diminish completely, but it will ebb until effective stimulation is reinstated. Effective stimulation can be anything that arouses you. If it doesn't arouse you, it is obviously not effective for you. Consequently, you may be very turned on by manual or oral stimulation before intercourse and feel very close to having an orgasm, but once intercourse starts, and the focus shifts to vaginal stimulation, you may experience a drop in the level of arousal. Although you may enjoy the physical and psychological experience of intercourse, you may not be able to reach orgasm this way. Women who have had a number of experiences of this nature may find themselves turning off when intercourse begins because they have learned to equate intercourse with the end of the more intense stimulation.

Effective stimulation is generally required up to and during the orgasm; if stimulation is discontinued during the orgasm itself, the orgasm may stop abruptly before completion. This incomplete release can be an intensely frustrating and unsatisfying experience. So let me repeat: consistent, continuous stimulation of a type dictated by individual preference is required to bring a woman to orgasm.

Women's experience of orgasm tends to vary. Orgasm has been described as a "rush," "a mint-flavored heat wave," like "one heartbeat all over," or a "misty cloud that envelops me." Marion describes her orgasm as "this pleasurable thing that flows over me and I feel like I'm flowing down a river—feeling warmth, and for a short time I lose all thoughts of everything." Gloria has a different experience. She says, "I sort of feel this feeling—I feel this buildup, then there is this feeling after it that's different, that's distinct—and I don't feel contractions, but I don't feel like going on anymore. And I feel relaxed."

The resolution phase describes the return of the sexual organs back to their accustomed resting state. The swelling of the areolas subsides, and as a result the nipples may appear even more erect. If a sex flush occurred, it now disappears. Sometimes a fine film of perspiration appears over the body. There is general relaxation of muscular tension. The uterus and clitoris return to their normal resting positions. Some women experience a soreness of the clitoral area for a few moments after orgasm. The vagina returns from its ballooned state back to being a potential space.

This return to the normal, unstimulated state may be completed within a few moments to half an hour after the occurrence of orgasm. If orgasm does not occur, the resolution phase can take an hour or longer. The length of time required for the completion of the resolution phase will usually be determined by the level of arousal attained during the plateau phase. The greater the arousal, the longer the time required for resolution. Women sometimes complain that increased congestion of blood in the pelvic region may leave them feeling bloated and uncomfortable when orgasm has not occurred. This feeling of discomfort may last for several hours after sexual stimulation has been discontinued.

Some women are capable of being stimulated to orgasm again before the resolution phase has been completed. Women with this capacity have been labeled "multiply orgasmic." Most men require periods of time ranging from a few seconds or minutes, usually in young men, to thirty minutes or several hours or even days in older men before they are capable of a new erection and subsequent ejaculation.[15] Some women do not seem to experience any such refractory period, whereas other women do seem to have a normal refractory period of some duration before they are capable of a second or third orgasm; other women feel complete after one orgasm. The response may also vary depending upon circumstances.

When Kinsey first published *Sexual Behavior in the Human Female* in 1953, a great furor took place over his disclosure that 14 percent of the women he interviewed claimed they were regularly capable of responding orgasmically two, three, and even more times during one sexual encounter.[16] Critics claimed that this was an impossibility and that Kinsey had been taken in, and these women were really frigid.[17] Masters and Johnson have subsequently found that some women are capable of more than one orgasm within a fairly short period of time if continually stimulated.[18] However, an innate capability may bear no relation to what is satisfying for the individual woman. You may be content with one orgasm or have two on rare occasions. Perhaps if you have any more than that, you may find the process more unpleasant than rewarding. On the other hand, you may be capable of experiencing and enjoying a number of orgasms in sequence. Regrettably, the recent emphasis on multiple orgasms has made many women feel inferior or inadequate if they prefer to experience only one orgasm. And this expectation adds a tremendous burden to the woman who rarely, if ever, experiences orgasm and now is expected to have three or four.

What is important is the woman's own pattern and her satisfaction with it. Some women reach orgasm quickly, while others respond more slowly. Many women have one strong orgasm, others have a number of mild ones, and many levels exist between the two extremes. In some women the first orgasm is strongest and the rest are milder; or the first is the mild one, the second more intense, and if there are more, they may vary in intensity. What fits for you may not fit for your friend. One way of responding is not innately superior to any other. However, people often think that "the grass is always greener" elsewhere. We expect that what we don't experience is really better than what we do experience. One can certainly remain dissatisfied and disappointed if one wants to, especially since there is no way to experience what someone else experiences internally. However, the investigation of options (see Chapter 9) with no expectations can be a way to explore the range of your orgasm, but enjoying your own sexual response and being comfortable with that response is essential.

Many of us have difficulty identifying whether or not we have had an orgasm. We've been told, "You'll know it if you've had it." If we don't know it for sure, we figure we haven't. We look for signposts. Do we have a sex flush? Can we feel any vaginal contractions? Does our clitoris swell? Do our nipples look erect afterward? However, physiological signs are not the measure of a subjective experience. Perhaps you don't know if you're having orgasms because you're looking for the wrong signposts. Do you end up feeling relaxed—not exhausted, but relaxed? When you masturbate, when do you choose to stop? Because you're frustrated? Because you've set aside a specific amount of time and it's over? Or because you feel satisfied and feel no need to continue? Feelings of satisfaction, relaxation, and a warm glow are the signs to look for, whether or not contractions, nipple erection, and sex flush are present or noticeable.

The following are some descriptions of the sexual arousal and release process. Harriet writes:

Not having had an orgasm until I was an adult influenced what I thought orgasm was. Finally achieving orgasm was a tremendous positive experience, but the sensation of orgasm itself was fleeting, not as earth-shaking or powerful as I had anticipated. More frequently experiencing orgasm has shown me they vary considerably in intensity, duration, type of contractions, and thoughts leading up to it. For me orgasm is a wonderful pleasure. My body feels very powerful and I feel powerful enough to face problems that seem insuperable. Let me describe my orgasm on two levels . . . my mind and my body. My mind anticipates the future relaxation as my imagination savors the release of tension. Then, as I begin to stimulate myself, my body takes over. I concentrate very hard on not losing the good feelings of sexual tension focusing mostly in my pelvis, but all over my body. As the stimulation continues I feel rich, warmer and warmer, more and more myself. Suddenly I feel only in the clitoral area and feel as if I want to suck with my whole body. Thoughts are there, but they are second to feelings like a magnificent animal. Then contractions begin and sometimes end quickly or continue. As they end, the orgasm is over suddenly. I feel so good yet often wish it had lasted longer. Usually my tension is gone and I can sleep refreshed, but sometimes thoughts take over again. My orgasms make me feel more myself than any other single experience. They are pure power and pleasure.

Carol expresses her experience this way:

In an orgasm I tense my muscles, my feet and hands, grimace, my middle (torso) convulses. Then I feel lightness in my head and a relaxing warm feeling. The feeling is one of well-being, spent.

Kelly uses a beautiful image to describe her experience:

> As soon as I begin rubbing my clitoris I get a pleasant tick-lish feeling, and whenever I hit an especially sensitive spot, my whole body jerks slightly. After five to ten minutes of rubbing, a new sensation takes over, and I know I am about to have an orgasm.
>
> The best analogy I can use to describe this new sensation is that I am standing on a deserted beach watching a tremendous wave on the horizon coming toward me. This wave gradually comes closer and closer and becomes bigger and bigger until it reaches me and washes over me. As the wave actually hits me, I reach orgasm and a graph of that sensation would be similar in shape to an open umbrella. At the most intense seconds of orgasm, I feel as if I am going up along the shaft of the umbrella and when I reach the point of the umbrella, I feel as if I am coming back down on all sides of the open umbrella. Afterward, I feel very tired and relaxed, and in ten minutes or so I feel ready to start again.

Primed with this information about your genitals and the way in which the sexual response cycle proceeds, you can learn about your responses by first becoming familiar with your own genitals.

Spend half an hour carefully examining your genitals with a hand mirror. If you feel uncomfortable doing this, spend only a few seconds looking at your genitals in a dim light. Then, build up the time and the intensity of the light until you have examined all the structures carefully. Label the parts of that special place (using the illustrations on Page 49 as a guide). By touching all the areas with your fingers, see if you can deter-mine any differences in sensitivity. Notice the colors and tex-tures of the areas. Place your fingers inside your vagina both to feel the pubococcygeal muscle that surrounds the opening and to see if some areas are more sensitive to touch than others. Some women find pressure placed against the front part of the vagina most pleasurable. Other women are more responsive on the right, the left, or the area closest to the anus. Do you notice any differences? No part is likely to be very sensitive until you are more sexually aroused, so don't be concerned if you don't feel much at first. Later, as you begin to explore more intensely, the differences will become more apparent, although you may find that sensations vary from time to time. In any case, the more familiar you are with your own genitals, the easier it will be for you to share them with your lover in a comfortable and self-accepting way. It is important to examine your own genitals carefully and locate all the structures. It is interesting that although we have examined most of the other areas of our bodies, few of us have ever looked closely at our genitals. By not examining this area, we perpetuate the mystery of sexuality and prevent ourselves from really understanding how our genitals work. When I suggested to one group that they examine their genitals at home, Sherry was stunned. She had been planning a visit to the doctor to find out if she had clitoral adhesions. The idea of exploring her own genitals had never occurred to her.

Some women expect to find their genitals ugly and disgusting. Given society's stress on cleanliness, we may have been made to feel embarrassed because our genitals are damp and have a slight but distinct natural odor. But there is no reason for us to feel ashamed. The advertising industry has offered us deodorant sprays to keep the genitals dry and sweet smelling. These sprays can cause more harm than good. Women have found that some of these sprays can irritate the very sensitive membranes of this area and cause considerable discomfort.[19] Similarly, washing your genitals too thoroughly with soap, especially deodorant soap, can also cause irritations or vaginal infections. The best solution is to wash the genital area thoroughly and regularly with warm water, especially if you're prone to gynecological problems. If there is no infection present, the genital area will have no more than a slight, natural odor.

Once you have examined your body and your genitals carefully and completely, we can move on. There is more to orgasm than just physiology. What is happening up in our heads is at least as important as what is taking place in the pelvic region.

6: Psychological Aspects of Reaching Orgasm

Sexual arousal consists of more than just physical genital stimulation. Genital stimulation is usually necessary for producing a satisfying and orgasmic sexual experience, but all the stimulation in the world may not produce an orgasm if desire is absent or your attention is elsewhere. If your mind is focused on sexual sensation, your body can enjoy it more fully. Outside distractions, anxiety, or anger operate to divert attention from sexual pleasure and can end up diluting the sexual experience.

If you're angry at your partner and don't want to have an orgasm; if you're afraid or uncomfortable in the sexual situation; if you're tired from a long, hard day; if you've been immersed in your work and can't get it off your mind; if the children cry in the next room or if the telephone rings; or if you're preoccupied with other thoughts, your mind may prevent your body from experiencing orgasm. These distinctions will not necessarily prevent you from enjoying the sexual encounter, but they can block your ability to respond orgasmically.

In one of the group sessions, Harriet recalled that she was able to respond to the point of orgasm more quickly if, before she began lovemaking, she checked to make sure the children were asleep, the front entrance light was out, and the telephone was off the hook. Having removed these possible causes of distraction, she could relax and enjoy the sexual stimulation more completely.

Kinsey,[1] Kaplan,[2] and Fisher,[3] all refer to distractions, fatigue, and preoccupation as being the most pervasive barriers to a woman's enjoyment of a satisfactory sexual experience. But there are some distractions that may not be obvious. Interruptions in lovemaking for a cigarette or sip of wine can lower your level of general arousal. Or, you may turn on some music to enhance lovemaking only to find that it does the opposite.

Sally found that the music she chose to play while masturbating interfered with sexual arousal. She would get so involved humming the songs and singing the words that she would forget about the sexual feelings. Women differ in the way they respond to sounds. Some women find that some sounds help build sexual excitement. Connie found that when she heard her children calling, she knew that she had to have an orgasm now or never and just knowing that helped her reach a climax.

There are techniques that you can use to overcome the diverting effect of outside distractions if you are susceptible to them. "White noise," a constant drone of undifferentiated and monotonous sound, such as running water, a fan, a hair dryer, or vibrator, may help to relax both partners and drown out external distractions—as might the record *Environments*, which has the sound of the ocean roaring on one side and birds singing on the other.

Relaxation, the use of fantasy, erotica, and focusing attention on the physical sensations work as mental aphrodisiacs to block external distractions while acting as a sort of lubricant that helps to get sensual and sexual messages flowing.

Erotic stimuli, or "mental or psychological aphrodisiacs," are psychological inputs that help to put you in a sexual mood and keep you there. A romantic candlelight dinner or quiet talking in front of a roaring fire can be arousing preludes to sex. Pictorial representations of naked men or women, erotic films, and written erotica that explicitly describe sexual activities are helpful to some women. During sex you might find that concentrating on memories of past erotic episodes or fantasies of sexual activities you might or might not ever perform or the visual input of your lover's nude or semi-nude body may aid in keeping you focused. Attending to these psychological aphrodisiacs can help orient your mind and body, your total self, toward sexual pleasure.

In the 1940s, Kinsey found considerable differences between a man's ability and a woman's ability to use fantasy, visual erotic stimuli, and written erotica as sexual enhancements. Men were far more responsive to these mental aphrodisiacs while women tended to respond more readily to romantic rather than explicitly sexual stimuli.[4] A dozen roses, a loving champagne toast, or light body stroking accompanied by passionate kissing may be as sexually stimulating, or more stimulating for women, than thinking about intercourse or actually engaging in it. Exclusive dependence on romantic stimuli for sexual arousal may produce some problems, however. First of all, it may not always be possible to plan ahead and prepare a romantic scene. Sexual desire may arise on the spur of the moment, possibly just from the comfort and warmth of your lover's body lying next to yours. Secondly, roses may put you in the proper frame of mind for sex, but more explicit sexual stimuli may be necessary for orgasm.

According to more recent research, the above-mentioned differences in response to erotic stimuli appear to be more a result of early conditioning than an innate difference in psychological makeup between men and women. The Playboy

Foundation Study found that "women today are far more likely to be aroused by erotic materials and fantasies . . . than was true only a generation ago."[5] A study done by Schmidt and Sigusch with "relatively sexually emancipated" and sexually experienced college students at the University of Hamburg showed no significant difference between the response of young men and young women to erotic material, both visual and written. Although, overall, the men reported feeling slightly more aroused than the women.[6]

These results indicate that it is possible, if not probable, that women can, perhaps with broadened experience, recondition themselves to respond positively to erotic stimuli. In fact, many women in the groups found this to be true. Women who had never been exposed to either graphic or written erotica, and had never used fantasy as an adjunct to sexual stimulation either while alone or with a partner, began to experiment. Several women found sexually explicit movies and novels highly stimulating. Others have been able to fantasize sexual scenes that were very erotic to them. Fantasy did not always come easily initially, but some of the women became more and more able to develop their imaginative abilities in this direction, with very rewarding results.

Feeling sexual and erotic in your mind as well as your body is important to orgasmic release. Retraining yourself to be more erotically responsive means experimenting for a while until you can tell which particular modes of erotic stimulation you find most arousing. The three most common mental aphrodisiacs used by women are: fantasy, erotica (both written and graphic), and total concentration on the pleasurable sensations occurring throughout the body, especially in the genital area.

A major advantage of fantasy as an aid to physical sexual stimulation is that it requires no equipment and is always available. Most of us have been endowed with minds that are creative enough to manufacture fantasies out of thin air. We all do some daydreaming. We may have fantasized about getting to know a handsome man we passed walking down a street; about getting a new job or promotion that may be imminent or only remotely possible; or about the vacation that doesn't begin for another two months. Before getting married, how many of us have fantasized about our futures? These and many other fantasies occupy some of our free time as we relax and let our minds wander; they are acceptable fantasies. Still, many women feel guilty if their fantasies become sexually explicit. We have been so well trained to think anything sexual is unacceptable that we may feel guilty—either promiscuous or oversexed—if these thoughts enter our minds, and many of us may fiercely guard against their occurrence.

Since women rarely share sexual fantasies with one another, we have little with which to compare and contrast fabrications. *My Secret Garden* and *Forbidden Flowers* by Nancy Friday are not scientifically documented accounts of female fantasies, but rather interesting compilations of fantasies reported to the author by various women. These books give an idea of what fantasies of other, very normal women, are like. They may help you to accept your own fantasies and to be less judgmental about them. They may also give you some themes to incorporate into your own fantasy life.

A fantasy is simply a mental creation. A marvelous quality of the human mind is that it has many levels of awareness. Dreams arise out of our subconscious. Our conscious minds direct everyday life. The imaginative function is in between— under our control, but not totally real—where we can create our own thoughts for the pleasure that they produce. Combining the pleasure of the mind with the pleasure of the physical senses can result in a more intensely enjoyable sexual experience. Fantasy can be fun and, like dreaming, provides a release for the tensions produced by our lives. We can spend our time and energy analyzing our fantasies if we want to, or we can simply enjoy them.

Having a fantasy does not mean you will want to act it out in reality. As a matter of fact, in the women's groups we have found that by giving women "permission" to enjoy and indulge their fantasizing abilities, they actually become less afraid that they will act out these impulses unless they consciously choose to do so.

Even though fantasy is a natural and normal activity, many women who fantasize while masturbating or during sex with a partner may feel guilty. This guilt usually has more to do with the content of the fantasies than with the actual act of fantasizing itself. We can experience guilt either because of the sexual acts we imagine performing, or the people we choose as fantasy partners.

A very common concern centers around the identity of the people with whom, in our fantasies, we are sexually involved. If the imagined lover is a woman, some heterosexual women fear they may be latent homosexuals. However, lesbian fantasies are not uncommon among heterosexual women, just as lesbians may fantasize about male lovers. Women are attractive and erotic beings. An aroused woman is sexually exciting. Many of us wonder what sex is like for two women together even when we may have no real desire for a lesbian relationship. It is only natural to allow in thought the things one might not feel comfortable expressing in real life. After all, two women who are both comfortable expressing their sexual feelings to each other will find their lovemaking just as erotic and exciting as a man and a woman find theirs. Through fantasy one is free to explore the whole gamut of human sexual expression.

Women commonly experience concern when the lover in

the fantasy is not the real lover or husband of the woman who is enjoying the fantasy. He may be a friend, a boss, an acquaintance, a stranger, or even a relative. Carmen felt terribly guilty because her fantasies during masturbation and even during actual lovemaking with her lover involved other men. She agonized about her fantasies because she considered absolute sexual fidelity a must in a meaningful relationship. She felt she was unfaithful because her thoughts were of other men, even though she had no intention or even any real desire to sleep with the men in her fantasies. She became more comfortable when she realized that her mind was allowing her the variety that was totally unacceptable to her in reality, especially when she saw that she did not act on her fantasies.

Often we don't allow ourselves the freedom to fantasize during lovemaking because we feel this must mean we do not find our partner sufficient. Darlene had been married for twenty-five years but still felt guilty if the mere sight of her husband undressed did not turn her on. She felt that her love for him should in itself make his nudity automatically arousing to her. In actuality human beings do not respond in this fashion. In time we become used to seeing our partner naked, and nakedness is no longer linked only to sexuality.

Fantasizing about other men or women cannot be interpreted as proof that we are tired of our real-life lover. Ask your male partner if he ever fantasizes about other women when he is making love to you. Most men will tell you that, on occasion, they do fantasize about other women or previous sexual experiences, something that adds to their enjoyment while taking nothing away from yours. If we accept fantasy while making love or at other times as a perfectly healthy and natural experience, it can serve us well.

Some women confide their fantasies to their partners and sometimes they keep them entirely to themselves. Many couples find swapping fantasies during lovemaking very stimulating. If you think you might enjoy sharing your fantasy life with your partner, you might ask him how he feels about it first and act accordingly.

The most common detrimental effect of fantasy occurs when women conclude that they must be perverted if their fantasies contain any unusual sexual acts. In reality, many fantasies contain elements of what some would consider perverse. For example, some of the most common themes in the fantasies of women revolve around rape or forceful seduction. Generally, the woman fantasizing is being taken by force and required to submit to the desires of her seducer/rapist. Guilt is triggered by the fact that the woman is enjoying the rape and is becoming highly aroused while imagining it. This, of course, conflicts with her intellectual awareness that she should not enjoy this form of sexuality. Actually, if she were really being raped she would probably not enjoy it. However, in the fantasy, she is safe and in charge. Her arousal stems from the fact that the man is so taken with her, he cannot restrain himself. The act is one of passion, not violence.

A second common theme that may cause women distress is the reverse of the last theme. In these fantasies, it is the woman who is the aggressor and her partner is a mere servant or slave who is there only to administer to her needs and desires. She takes all the pleasure and gives nothing in return. Beth experienced considerable self-loathing because she always appeared to need this fantasy to reach orgasm. She said, "The men in my sexual fantasies have no meaning to me. They are there solely to give me pleasure. As I become sexually excited, I zero in on my own feelings and nothing else is important to me. My lover is an object who is there solely to create the sexual feelings. He feels nothing for me and I nothing for him. I end up feeling worthless because he is so cool and uninvolved with me and I have been so inconsiderate of his needs." Beth had considerable trouble accepting her fantasies. She felt there was something perverted about her total concern with her own sexual feelings to the exclusion of all else. She felt selfish. However, once she gave herself permission to get into the fantasy wholeheartedly, to accept it and go along with it rather than fighting, succumbing, and feeling guilty, she began to feel better about that fantasy. She no longer wasted her energy on fighting the fantasy. She could allow herself to relax and enjoy the selfish feelings without feeling guilty, and soon she found she was able to become aroused through the use of other fantasies as well.

Scenes of orgies, mate swapping, or a *ménage à trois* are frequent fantasies. Scenes including animals and spanking, whipping, or other sadomasochistic acts are not uncommon either.[7] The numbers of different and diverse fantasies have led me to expect the unexpected, and I have found no particular connection between the type of fantasy and the personality of the woman.

It seems only natural that we should imagine the illicit during sexual fantasy, for hasn't sex and everything associated with it always been somehow illicit? Try to stop psychoanalyzing your fantasies. Instead, enjoy the fantasy fully and freely and see if anything changes for you. Also, fantasies evolve over time. What you find exciting this month may become mundane as you explore new and different sexual turn-ons. Fantasy is clearly one of the ways you can widen your sexual experiences without actually indulging in acts that may be unacceptable to you. It is also a very positive way to focus your mind during sexual activity so that you can concentrate completely on sexual pleasure.

Not all of us have the ability to fantasize with ease at the beginning, and few of us will ever experience an orgasm by fantasy alone, but you may be able to develop the ability to fantasize, which may greatly enhance your sexual experiences.

Erotica—literature, pictures, or movies—can be potent mental aphrodisiacs, but they are not frequently indulged in by most women. Traditionally, pornography has been created by men to appeal to masculine tastes, and written accounts of sexual activities are frequently inaccurate as far as female sexuality is concerned.

Many erotic films or erotic photographs may fail to appeal to women, partially because the fantasies portrayed in them are likely to be male fantasies that exploit the female. Women are depicted as perfect bodies, but nothing more. Also, women were taught not to respond to explicitly sexual pictures and movies. At best, pornography was something indulged in by college men at bachelor parties and at worst by drunken lechers in sordid theaters. Many women, when exposed for the first time to hard-core pornography, either written or graphic, are taken aback or overcome with embarrassment or disgust. Many of the women I have worked with responded to their first experiences with pornography with intense laughter. Mostly because of their embarrassment, very few reacted at first with sexual arousal. If one is trained to believe that displays of sexuality are perverted and distasteful, one responds accordingly. Janice saw a pornographic movie for the first time and was very uptight and uncomfortable during the showing. She claimed, "I hated the film, but couldn't wait to hop into bed afterward." In retrospect, she thought she was probably more turned on by the film than anyone else in the audience, even though she was not aware of these feelings at the time. However, despite the constraints I have described, many women can now allow themselves to feel turned on and enjoy erotic films—especially since films like *Cabin Fever, The Voyeur,* and *The Hottest Bid* have been designed specifically to appeal to women and couples.[8]

Considerable misunderstanding and hurt feelings can result from attitudinal differences between men and women about visual stimuli. Many males don't understand why their female lovers do not respond to the display of the male body and genitals. The lack of positive response from a female partner may lead the male to feel rejected and question her love for him. Meanwhile, the female may consider his display distasteful and may think him perverted or vulgar. Similarly, many women take offense when their male lover seeks additional stimulation through pornographic materials. A woman may wonder why her male partner is not sexually satisfied with her alone and may fear he is losing interest in her. The male partner, on the other hand, cannot comprehend why she is not similarly aroused by the pornographic material. Open discussions with your partner about the things you find erotically stimulating can be very enlightening. It is important to recognize existing differences so that these differences do not cause hurt feelings and rifts in an otherwise positive and happy relationship. Just because you state where you are now doesn't mean you have to stay there. You can slowly broaden your experience if you wish to.

The difference in male and female response to written erotic material is similar to the difference in response to graphic sexual portrayals. In general women seem to respond more positively to love stories than they do to more explicit depictions of the sex act. Again, this may be the result of early conditioning. It used to take Jane one and a half hours of constant genital stimulation with a vibrator before she could have an orgasm. In the group we suggested that the women experiment with some erotic novels while masturbating. Jane came back in the next session reporting that with the aid of the erotica, she could have an orgasm in ten minutes or less. The same results have been reported by other women who required a tremendous length of time to reach orgasm either manually or through the use of a vibrator. This is not to say that your goal should be to have an orgasm as quickly as possible, but if you require over an hour of constant clitoral and genital stimulation, it's very likely that your head is elsewhere. Reading erotica can help to block out other distracting thoughts and worries while keeping your mind focused on the sexual stimulation.

It is easy to see how erotic material can be read while masturbating, but it might be more difficult to see how it can be used with lovemaking. There are many ways to incorporate erotica into partner sex. Reading to each other can be arousing or reading together silently can put you in the mood for sex. One person can read aloud while the other can engage in body caressing and other physical stimulation.

As with other accompaniments to sex, a frequent fear is that the use of erotica is abnormal or perverted, that one becomes addicted to using this method and will not be able to make love without it. But there is nothing more perverted or abnormal about using fantasy or erotica to enhance sex than there is in using a special perfume or a sexy negligee. They can all enrich the lovemaking. The major difference is that the use of perfume and negligee appears to be more acceptable to society. But really, your sex life is private and no one except your partner need approve of the things you like to do while making love.

Some women are prevented from experimenting with pornography by their reluctance to go into a store and buy it. Certainly walking into an "adult" bookstore in a sleazy part of town may present a disagreeable experience. Most women feel embarrassed; you may be the only woman in the store. But if you watch the men, it turns out that they are equally embarrassed, if not more so by your presence, and will turn their backs to the aisle and bury their heads in their magazines as you walk by. You need not confront the "adult" bookstore, however, because vast amounts of erotic material are available in regular bookstores. I myself have edited four volumes of erotic stories especially written for women and couples. Women wrote about their real sexual experiences in *Pleasures* and about their fantasies in *Erotic Interludes*. I compared erotica written by men and women in *The Erotic Edge* and *Seductions*.

Different types of erotica appeal to different women. Some like flowery words and descriptions, while others prefer four-letter words. Jenny claimed that the "nastier" the novel the more she liked it. If you try reading erotica a few times and find that it does nothing for you, then you can reject it. But if you've never really experienced it, how do you know for sure?

Unquestionably women can appreciate mental aphrodisiacs, but it may just entail time and experimentation to acquire a taste for something new. There are few non-Greeks who immediately love the taste of retsina, a resinated Greek wine, but after a few attempts at drinking it, it becomes familiar and much more pleasant. Soon the taste may become so enjoyable and distinct that unresinated wine, though good, may seem dull in comparison. Then again, some people never develop a taste for retsina and prefer another type of wine. The same is true of the erotic adjuncts to sex. It may take time to develop a taste for some of them or all of them, but there is a good chance they can enhance your sexuality if you take the time to experiment with them.

Another way to occupy your mind with sexual thoughts so you don't get distracted by nonsexual things while making love is by focusing on the physical stimulation. For example, to really feel the sensations in your breasts as they are being kissed and massaged. Concentrating closely on the good feelings can block out all other thoughts and outside distractions. Ellen said that when she experienced her first orgasm, it felt like her clitoris was almost at her chin, she was concentrating on it so hard.

According to Kinsey 36 percent of the women who masturbated used nothing more than physical stimulation to have an orgasm.[9] If you don't fantasize easily and pornography just doesn't turn you on, try concentrating very carefully on the tactile sensations. Some women enjoy being rubbed with oil, feathers, leather, etc. So we can capitalize on this responsiveness to physical stimulation by really exploring it and focusing on it.

Alcohol and certain tranquilizers can have a disinhibiting effect on some women. Evelyn says that having a few glasses of wine before making love not only helps to relax her, but as with other alcoholic drinks, makes her less self-conscious. She becomes more assertive and feels greater freedom to express her sexuality.

Alcohol and tranquilizers are similar in that a small amount can enhance sexuality while a large amount can lower sexual excitability.[10] Too much of either can result in sleep rather than passion, and there is no way to predetermine how much is too much for a particular individual. Some women can get high on a glass of wine and others don't feel a thing after several glasses of scotch. Through careful experimentation you can find out how much allows you to loosen up and how much pushes you into oblivion.

Marijuana can also enhance sexuality.[11] It can act to relax inhibitions in much the same way that alcohol does. However, some women have reported that their experience with pot is so concrete and literal that they cannot get beyond the feeling of skin rubbing on skin to enjoy the sexual sensations produced by the skin being rubbed.

You can try some of these aids on your own first with masturbation and then if and when you feel comfortable you can weave them into your shared lovemaking. Use your imagination. Take a risk and maybe try out some of your secret erotic fantasies or thoughts. As long as your partner is agreeable, no one else need be consulted. Probably the worst outcome would be uproarious laughter and possible disruption of the sexual mood. But with experimentation, you may discover things that enhance your sex life and which may even keep you feeling turned on for days.

What we are setting out to do is to free the mind to concentrate on sexual feelings. Putting your body in the right place is the first step. Putting your mind there, too, completes the picture.

7: Why Masturbation?

Masturbation is one of the best ways to learn about your sexual responses. Once you learn about how you respond—through stimulating yourself while free of outside distractions—you will be able to achieve more pleasure during lovemaking or teach your partner how to stimulate you to sexual pleasure and eventually to orgasm.

According to Kinsey, "Masturbation may be defined as deliberate self-stimulation which effects sexual arousal."[1] The stimulation can be direct manual stimulation of the genitals or other parts of the body; it can entail the use of objects other than the hand to effect arousal; it can be the result of muscular tension or just mental stimulation. The stimulation does not have to result in orgasm to be called masturbation.[2]

Of all sexual practices, masturbation is probably the most difficult to talk about. It is an intimate and very personal experience that we have been taught is dirty, sinful, shameful, even physically debilitating. The guilt, fear, anxiety, and repulsion that surrounds masturbation is astounding, especially when one realizes not only how pervasive it is among human beings, but how beneficial, pleasurable, and relaxing an experience it can be. Most important, from the standpoint of the pre-orgasmic woman, it is the surest, most effective way to achieve orgasmic release. Many women don't consider the orgasms they have with masturbation as being "real." They believe that "true orgasms" occur only during intercourse. But as was discussed in Chapter 5, all orgasms are real no matter how they are produced, although the total subjective experience may differ depending on the situation and mode of stimulation.

Sixty-two percent of the women Kinsey interviewed masturbated, and only 4 to 6 percent of these women masturbated without reaching orgasm.[3] The ones who did have orgasms were able to do so in 95 percent of their masturbatory experiences.[4] Hence, most women who masturbate enjoy orgasm through self-stimulation almost every time that they undertake to do so.

Overall, Kinsey found that "the type of premarital activity in which the female had acquired her experience did not appear to have been as important as the fact that she had or had not experienced orgasm."[5] Women who had experienced orgasm premaritally, through any means, were able to respond orgasmically with marital sex three times as often as women who had no orgasmic experience prior to marriage.[6] Masters and Johnson found that the orgasms produced by masturbation occurred more dependably, more rapidly, and were of greater intensity than those achieved through stimulation by a partner.[7] These are just a few of the statistics that support the value of masturbation as an excellent way to learn about your own sexuality, and to achieve orgasm.

The reason self-stimulation works so well to produce orgasm is that you are the only one involved. There is no one to distract you or for you to worry about pleasing. You can focus totally on yourself, take as much time as you need, and you don't need a partner who is willing to cooperate. You are the one in control, which has benefits. First of all, once you are free from being observed you can focus all your attention on the different kinds of touches, pressures, and positions. The immediate feedback provided by self-stimulation allows you to make the subtle changes necessary to meet your needs. If the feelings are getting too intense or uncomfortable, you can stop for a while, until you become more familiar with those feelings. You never have to go faster than is comfortable. Also, since one's first orgasms are frequently mild in intensity, you are more likely to recognize one when it occurs because orgasms with masturbation tend to be more intense.

If you are uncertain as to whether you have ever experienced orgasm or are certain that you haven't, masturbation can be the key to orgasmic discovery. After her group ended, Sherry said, "I have no doubt that if I hadn't masturbated, I would never have had an orgasm." Once you have learned to overcome your inhibitions and abandon yourself to the physical sensations of orgasm with masturbation, you may become more capable of responding in a similar way with your partner—if you want to. The successful experience of having orgasms with masturbation helps to build positive expectations of having more orgasms by yourself and eventually with a partner. If you choose to continue to hold back the orgasm you can do so, but at least you'll have the choice.

Contrary to popular belief, women do not get "hooked" on masturbation, thereby becoming incapable of having orgasms in any other way. Kinsey states, "We have seen very few cases of females who had encountered any difficulty with transferring their masturbatory experience to coitus, although we have seen some hundreds of cases of females who were considerably disturbed because they were unable to accomplish the anatomic impossibility of transferring their clitoral reactions to vaginal responses."[8]

According to Mary Jane Sherfey, "orgasm tends to increase pelvic vasocongestion; thus, the more orgasms achieved, the more can be achieved."[9] The more orgasms you have by any method—self-stimulation included—the more sexually responsive you are likely to become. The more you exercise and keep the muscles toned, the healthier and better functioning your body systems—including the sexual—will become.

Even if you achieve orgasm frequently, there are many good reasons to masturbate. For example, masturbation is always available including times when your partner isn't—either because you are physically separated or because your lover is not in the mood at the same time you are. Masturbation allows you to be sexually independent from a partner. Lack of a partner no longer means lack of sex. Your ability to produce your own orgasm can reduce pressure on your partner to perform. Compare this situation to eating. Sometimes you may be hungry when your partner isn't around; you might prefer to eat with him, but you wouldn't consider starving just so you could eat together. You can satisfy your hunger for food by yourself with a meal or a snack and you can still join your partner later on if you like. This is also true of sexual hunger.

In addition, there may be times when you don't feel like interacting with your partner, times when you would prefer to be totally self-engrossed, forget your partner's needs, and enjoy masturbation just for the relaxing satisfaction it provides you. If you are both self-sufficient, there is more freedom to express your own needs rather than having to adapt your sexual tempo to your partner's.

Masturbation is in no way a reflection on the adequacy of the couple's sexual relationship. It can enlarge your sex life, not restrict it. Furthermore, self-stimulation can afford you a sense of control and self-confidence while helping you to like and enjoy your body better. And it's fun—an easy way to feel good all over.

A 1994 study found that 63 percent of women masturbated to relieve sexual tension, 42 percent for physical pleasure, 32 percent to relax, 32 percent when their partner was unavailable, and smaller percentages for reasons such as to relieve boredom, help them to sleep, and to keep them safe from AIDS and STDs.[10]

Still, a reasonable proportion of women don't masturbate for a variety of reasons. During the 1800s many books were written by physicians describing the horrors of masturbation. David Cole Gordon, in a small book called *Self Love*,[11] describes the ways in which masturbation was said to be responsible for all the major social and medical ills.

Masturbation was alleged to cause warts on one's hands, hair on the palms of hands, blindness, acne, sterility, and deformed babies. It was deemed responsible for all sorts of psychological problems. The source of this belief is an interesting one. It appears that doctors observed institutionalized mental patients and found that they masturbated. Of course, it should be noted that because these people were institutionalized, no other sexual outlet was available. Bizarre as it may sound, these were the observations that led to the conclusion that masturbation was the cause of the lunacy.[12]

Early myths about the physical and psychological dangers of masturbation have been well ingrained. Davis noted that most women who discontinued masturbating did so due to their fear that it would cause mental and physical deterioration.[13] Ann began masturbating as the result of the group treatment program and developed a urinary tract infection. Her immediate reaction was to think that the masturbation had caused it. She asked her doctor about it, and the doctor replied with a laugh that *she* had never developed a urinary tract infection from masturbating.

Other common reasons that prevent women from masturbating include moral proscription, not being aware that women could do it, or not knowing how to do it.[14] Margaret Mead says, "The female child's genitals are less exposed, subject to less maternal manipulation and less self-manipulation."[15] Therefore, it is likely that female children may fail to discover that their sex organs are sensitive to pleasurable stimulation.

Other obstacles to masturbating stem from the partner and the social situation. Jenny was afraid to masturbate for fear that she would be so turned on by her body that she would only be attracted to other female bodies. Many women feel a sense of self-devaluation if they masturbate, because they assume that a woman resorts to masturbation only if she can't get anything better.

Many men feel threatened by the idea that women masturbate, especially with a vibrator. A man may feel that if his partner can be sexually fulfilled on her own, she will have no need for him. He often does not recognize the previously mentioned advantages that masturbation affords him. What is inferred is that masturbation will lower a woman's desire for sexual contact with a partner. One woman told her male gynecologist that she masturbated and he gently told her that it was bad for her because she was depriving her husband of the pleasure that was his. In reality, a study by Greenberg showed no statistically significant relationship between the frequency of masturbation and the frequency of intercourse among the women polled.[16] Most women who masturbate have enough sexual energy to allow for masturbation as well as sexual activity with a partner—just as their partners do.

A considerable number of women avoid masturbation because they consider it morally wrong. Several religious denominations have condemned masturbation, sometimes in the context of a broader condemnation of any sexual activity that is not aimed at reproduction, or because it reflects carnal as opposed to spiritual pursuits.[17] These moral grounds have been a prime factor in preventing numerous women from beginning to masturbate.[18] However, once a woman has discovered masturbation as a sexual release, evidence indicates that she will only rarely discontinue the practice because of religious condemnation. Instead, she is likely to continue masturbating while experiencing significant feelings of guilt.[19] Laumann, Gagnon, Michael, and Michaels found that almost half the females who masturbated felt guilty about it.[20]

Any possible harmful effects of masturbation come from the worry and concern women have about the abnormality of the activity rather than from the activity itself. According to Kinsey, ". . . some millions of the females in the United States, and a larger number of males, have had their self-assurance, their social efficiency, and sometimes their sexual adjustments in marriage needlessly damaged—not by their masturbation, but by the conflict between practice and moral codes. There is no other type of sexual activity that has worried so many women."[21]

It could hardly be expected that after reading these passages, you will automatically and magically lose all of the negative feelings you may have about masturbation. The first time that you contemplate it, you probably won't feel very comfortable with the idea that self-stimulation is a good thing for you. But the act itself, and the positive learning about your sexual self that can be derived may, in time, make you more comfortable with the idea.

Despite the substantial negative conditioning surrounding the act of masturbation, Hunt[22] and Kinsey[23] both obtained figures that showed that 60 to 65 percent of the women interviewed had masturbated at some time during their lives. Heterosexual petting is the form of sexual activity the largest number of females report participating in before marriage; coitus is the sexual activity most frequently performed after marriage; and masturbation is the second most common sexual activity that women engage in both before and after marriage.[24]

Females can stimulate themselves sexually in many ways. Most commonly, female masturbation consists of manipulating the clitoris, the inner lips, or the whole genital area or by simply creating pressure by exerting muscular tension of the thighs and buttocks. Other methods include running water directly on the clitoris, using a vibrator or douches, or rubbing the genitals against pillows, clothing, or other objects. Beth had always masturbated by exerting rhythmical and steady muscle pressure while on her stomach with a pillow between her legs. She could have an orgasm after about twenty seconds, but she was unable to transfer this technique to partner sex, since this position could not be used in lovemaking with a partner. She learned to masturbate manually, and then could experience orgasms with a partner.

Chapter 8 will help you discover how to reach orgasm through masturbation. The exercises are important. Chapter 9 is designed to help you develop and extend your sexuality with self-stimulation, and set the stage for transferring what you've learned to a partner relationship. Masturbation can be the first step in becoming orgasmic. Not only is it a pleasurable and natural activity, but also it provides effective tools for change which can be used later.

8: Exercises

If you follow the steps in this chapter carefully and closely, chances are excellent that you will be able to become orgasmic within several weeks of practice.

In Chapter 4 we discussed the necessity of setting aside time and a private comfortable space in which to develop your sexuality. Now is the time to do it. You'll have to establish different priorities in your life to make time for yourself. You may even have to give up something different each day of the week in order to find an hour to devote to your sexuality. If you don't assertively take the time for yourself, you're likely to find that the day has ended and there is no time left to practice. Days can slip by in this way unless you are determined to make the time for your exercises.

Pick a time when you're not too tired. Marion had difficulty making the time. She would do her sexual homework at one o'clock in the morning just as she was going to bed and would often fall asleep in the middle of practicing. Then she set different priorities. One day, instead of practicing her flute, she practiced her sexual exercises during that hour; another day she got up an hour early; and a third day, instead of making the elaborate dinner she had initially planned, she settled for a simple meal instead. During that week she realized that she had been having orgasms during those late-night sessions, but she had been too tired to recognize them.

I know that if you can take time for yourself, you'll feel better about yourself and others will feel better about you. Someone who is feeling good about herself is much more enjoyable to be around than someone who is always concerned that she is not doing enough. If you have children, feeling better about yourself will result in your being a better companion and model for them.

An hour a day, *every day*, should be set aside for two to five weeks if you want to reestablish the sexual connections that have been disconnected for all these years.

Once you have made the decision to find an hour each day, think about how you can feel in a more sensual mood. Your mood is important, so pick a time when you are at ease and your energy level is fairly high. Take a long shower or bath; bring some fresh flowers into the room, light some candles, or burn some incense. Do whatever will create a sensual scene for you. Pretend a lover is returning from a long trip and arrange the room in the kind of romantic setting you know you both would enjoy. Lie down and enjoy the time; one of your favorite lovers can be you.

Learning to express your full sexuality means starting from the beginning. In our culture achieving sexual ease and comfort does not come naturally, any more than learning to walk would if you had spent your early years contained in a small box. In order to learn to walk, you would have to get out of the box and learn to use your legs—crawling, standing, and then finally walking. In order to have orgasmic sexual experiences, you may have to learn about sexual stimulation from the beginning, in the comfortable setting you've designed for yourself. Don't rush things. You have lots of time. All you need is determination and practice. You have the right to an orgasm, for yourself, not to keep your partner from feeling inadequate as a lover; *you* deserve the pleasure that a satisfying sexual relationship can bring.

For now, concentrate on learning to have an orgasm on your own through self-stimulation. Later you can concentrate on transferring the orgasm to the partner relationship. Certainly you can continue to make love with your partner as frequently as you usually do, but during partner sex make certain that you *do not* reach orgasm. Don't even think about orgasm; just concentrate on the feelings that you do experience with lovemaking and leave the orgasm for the hour a day you spend with yourself. If you feel yourself approaching orgasm with your partner, keep yourself from going over the top.

If you have not already done the exercises in Chapters 4 and 5, begin with them. Examine your body thoroughly, visually and through touch, for that first hour. During your hour the next day, examine your genitals with a mirror and explore each area to see if you notice any difference in sensitivity or sensations in the various parts of the genital area. Don't forget the Kegel exercises.

The exercise for the third night is to begin the actual masturbation. You may need to use some oil—massage oil, baby oil, coconut oil, or even vegetable oil will do. Scented massage oils can add to your sensual experience, but be careful that the oil contains no alcohol, since alcohol can irritate the mucous membranes of the genitals.

Use oil, saliva, or the natural lubrication of the vagina to keep the genital tissues moist so that no irritation develops. Explore by stimulating the area with various types of strokes and pressures. What do very light feathery touches feel like? How about harder rubbing? Try massaging the clitoral area with your fingertips by making gentle but firm circular motions. Some women like to stimulate the glans of the clitoris directly, while others find this area too sensitive for direct touch and prefer to massage the surrounding areas above, below, or to the sides of the clitoris. Find out what feels best for you. Many women rub one finger back and forth over the clitoris with varying speeds and intensity. The clitoris can be massaged between the forefinger and middle finger, or you can stroke up and down the clitoral shaft. Many women enjoy having their fingers or something else in the vagina while the clitoris is being stimulated.

If you notice some irritation of the area, you may be rubbing the skin surface rather than the structures below. A deeper type of rubbing generally produces less irritation to the genitals; rub as though you were massaging a tense muscle and wanted to reach the knot below the skin. This stroke would be different from the type you would use if you had a skin irritation and were rubbing the surface with a cream. If you do rub too hard or irritate the area, try moving a little more slowly and begin with a lighter touch. Don't be concerned; the irritation will disappear within a few hours or a day at the most. It may take a day or two for the genital area to get used to this new stimulation.

Remember, you're on a fact-finding mission now. You're learning. Feel whatever there is to feel. Don't hold back in anticipation; don't measure your sensations. Instead, tune in to any feelings that you do experience and enjoy them. At first, you will probably feel very little, but continue, and take note of even small feelings. It is precisely these little feelings that later turn into greater ones, but only after considerable practice.

In our groups we found that women tend to get stymied at various stages in the process of self-stimulation. The most consistent initial difficulty is finding the time to practice. Women try masturbating once or twice for a short period of time and, feeling discouraged and guilty, conclude that there is no hope for them, that there must be an easier way—and they give up. Perhaps it's like the first time you tried to bake a cake; it probably burned. If you had never tried again, you would have been a failure at cake baking. Perhaps instead you tried several times, went through a few trials before your cake was even edible, but now, it's probably pretty good.

If you don't invest some real time in self-sexuality, you won't get any results. The time is your responsibility. For most women, getting in contact with their sexuality takes perseverance. Many women require an hour every day for two to five weeks, so if you don't feel anything during the first few days, stick with it. You have lots of time ahead of you.

Some women find that despite their intellectual acceptance of masturbation, self-stimulation produces feelings of disgust, shame, guilt, or embarrassment. Your early negative conditioning about masturbation can reassert itself while you're in the act of doing it. Angela felt very guilty. She would do her exercises in the bedroom, where there was a picture of her parents hanging on the wall. She felt as if she were being watched and felt extremely guilty. Finally she turned the picture around and subsequently felt a whole lot better. Abby first did the exercises under the covers because she was embarrassed. Sarah used a blindfold—and had her first orgasm. Janice was uncomfortable with the homework, but felt reassured when she told her husband prior to beginning the assignment, "At least I know there are five other gals in the Bay Area doing what I'm going to do tonight." The five others were in her group. You can be assured that there are many more than five other females masturbating at any given time in your town. Kelly's initial reaction was that it was bad and dirty to be touching her genitals with her hand, but she got over the feelings with time and practice, as did Carmen, who responded to the exercise assignment by asking us if we were sure there wasn't some other way for her to become orgasmic. At first, she didn't want to do the exercises, but after other women began reporting that they were feeling sensations they had never felt before—and after one woman had an orgasm—Carmen decided it might be good training. By the time the group had ended, Carmen was orgasmic and masturbation for its own sake was more than acceptable to her.

If you're still finding masturbation and the thought of it disagreeable and offensive, don't try to fight the feelings. Exaggerate them! While you are stimulating yourself, let yourself feel disgusted. Make disagreeable sounds and exaggerate the motions that offend you. Stay with the foolish or uncomfortable feelings. Exaggerating them for a couple of hours should help to neutralize any negative reaction to the exercise.

Another difficulty that may arise for many women is that they say they feel *nothing*, even after a number of days of consistent practice. If you are one of these women, let's compare with your expectations the feelings you label as "nothing." Are you really feeling nothing? Or are you just not feeling what you anticipated? Compare the feeling in your clitoris to that in your elbow. Any difference? A small difference? Good! Keep at it. Maybe you are expecting to experience something different from the feelings that you *are* having at this time. However, by constantly focusing on what is *not* there, you may be losing sight of the feelings that *do* exist for you. A good strategy is to concentrate on what *is* happening rather than on what is not happening. At the beginning, you are looking for information about yourself—*not* instant orgasm. Even negative information—discovering the things that don't turn you on—is important.

Involve other parts of your body, in addition to your genitals, in the sexual stimulation. Massage your inner thighs, breasts or nipples, or other erotically sensitive areas with one hand as you stimulate the genital area with the other. Stimulate sensitive areas in the manner that feels best to you. You, and you alone, know what is most exciting and pleasurable for you. You are engaged in becoming the expert on yourself so explore a bit until you discover what feels best.

Don't forget the mental aphrodisiacs. Erotic writings, pictures or films, and fantasies can help take your mind off the cares of the day and focus it on the sensual feelings. Edna had her first orgasm after returning from seeing her first erotic movie.

Many women enjoy the "most patient lover" fantasy. Pretend that you are making love and your lover is infinitely patient. Your lover is willing to do anything and everything for you. A second enjoyable fantasy might be to imagine yourself as the world's most sensuous woman who is teaching an inexperienced lover the art of pleasing a woman.

Using muscular tension by rhythmically contracting the muscles in the pelvic and thigh region, or doing the Kegels while stimulating the clitoral area manually, can enhance your pleasure. A glass of wine or a martini might relax you for your hour so that you are better able to concentrate on the good feelings. If you find that your mind wanders while you are masturbating, take some time off to think about various nonerotic things. We all need some time to daydream, so acknowledge that need. Spend fifteen minutes just letting your imagination roam freely, and you may find that after that time you are more ready to attune your mind to sexual, sensual thoughts.

Let yourself go. Experiment. Darlene found it a turn-on to do the exercises while partially clothed. She said she felt like a dancer in a burlesque show and the thought really enhanced her sexual mood. Also, remember that music may either intensify arousal, or interfere with it.

To reach orgasm takes time, practice, and the right mental

attitude. Without the support of a group it might be a little more difficult, but don't get discouraged. If you feel as though you don't want to go on, then take a break. Many people find the exercises really enjoyable, so if you're finding them a chore or if you're spending the time but hating it, discontinue them for a day or two. Then resume the exercises when the pressure is off. Katie was really discouraged. She came to the group crying and just about ready to give up. She had only experienced two small sensations over the previous days of homework, and she wasn't even sure that she knew where her clitoris was. We told her to stimulate herself using a mirror so she could see where she was touching. It was clear that she was trying too hard and not enjoying it enough. She was looking for headlines and not paying sufficient attention to the fine print. Four days later she arrived exuberant, having discovered her first orgasm. After the group ended, Katie offered to come into other groups and tell them about her success story. She was twenty-six years old and had never had a single sexual feeling in her life. Now she was having orgasms and couldn't believe it.

You might find that, without the aid of group support to make you stick with it, you can come up with all sorts of ways to procrastinate. Here are some of the common problems I have heard from the women in the groups, and also ways to solve them. Perhaps by recognizing them you can devise ways to get beyond the typical initial resistance. If you've never masturbated before, your natural urges have probably been blocked by factors in your background. Overcoming these factors means sticking with the exercises even though you may find the task difficult at the beginning.

Evelyn complained that her hand got tired, so we suggested more movement of the fingers and less of the whole arm or vice versa depending upon the muscles that were being affected. If this problem persists, cut the exercise time down to half an hour and add five minutes to your time with each succeeding day until you are spending the full hour. It's very common for women to require an hour or even two hours of stimulation before that first orgasm occurs. Having an orgasm is like learning a new dance. If you don't get it right the first time and give up, you'll never learn. It takes time and practice.

Margaret would do the exercises for fifteen seconds while reading erotica and then would get so involved in the reading that she would forget about the manual stimulation. Remember that discontinuing the physical stimulation in females usually lowers the level of sexual arousal. To experience your first orgasm, it is important to keep your level of physical arousal high.

If this process is going to work, you have to really want the orgasm. If you don't think it worth the effort or if you don't expect results, you will probably be the victim of a self-fulfilling prophecy. Because you don't really try, it will fail. Things won't have changed and you still won't be orgasmic. But what would happen if you *really* tried? Cindy procrastinated by saying that since she had learned the information now, she would work on it later. "But when is later?" I asked her. She could have put it off forever without doing anything about it unless she set some goals right then. She began to see my point, but having that first orgasm was still a scary prospect for her. However, she thought it was worth it, and in the long run she recognized her fear and confronted it. Eve realized that setting aside time was essential, although she had difficulty making an hour's space for herself. She found it took her an hour just to get aroused. If she spent less time, she didn't seem to get anywhere.

One of the group leaders, Ms. Jeremy Brav, told a wonderful story as the women sat in a circle and talked about their experiences with the homework exercises. "Sometimes," she said, "I feel like we are all Indian ladies sitting around the campfire. We are trying to figure out how to allow the Great Spirit of the Orgasm to visit us. We can't *make* the Spirit come; it will come of its own accord. But through the years, lore has been handed down and we pass it around while we're waiting. Try this. Well, maybe this will make it come. And lo and behold the lore must work because the Great Spirit of the Orgasm does descend to grace us."

If you've been practicing the exercises for an hour a day for about ten days to two weeks and still aren't getting aroused (I don't mean not having orgasms, I mean not having any sexual feelings at all), there are some nonmanual techniques that may be just what you need to awaken your sexual feelings. I don't recommend using these techniques at the outset because I've found that it is better for women to touch themselves directly, to become comfortable with the genital area and get used to their bodies and their sexual feelings.

A vibrator or running water is a good addition to manual masturbation. It might make good sense to begin with manual stimulation and then after about ten to fifteen minutes employ another technique. Or, use one method one day and another the next day.

Many children discover the running water or bathtub technique. It consists of lying in the tub and maneuvering your body so that your genitals are directly under the faucet (this may not be physically possible given the shape of your body and the design of your tub); or attach a small hose to the faucet. Direct the stream of warm water onto the clitoral area. The sensation produced is akin to that of a thousand tiny fingers rapidly moving over the genitals. The pressure of the water on this sexually sensitive area can produce an orgasm. I say "can" because, as with other types of stimulation, it is possible mentally to fight the orgasm and prohibit it from happening, despite the effectiveness of the physical stimulation.

It is best to get used to the sensations gradually. Stay under the water for a while and then move away when you begin feeling sensations that are unfamiliar to you. Then move under again as you gradually become more comfortable with these new feelings. Leslie began experiencing orgasms this way and used to joke about how shriveled her skin was getting from taking so many baths.

Many types of vibrator/massagers are available at most drug and department stores. They can also be ordered by mail.[1] An electric one is generally preferable. The inexpensive battery-operated massagers are fine for some women, but many complain that they are noisier than the electric ones. Heating elements do not seem to be important, but a massager equipped with a variety of attachments can afford the versatility required for individual preferences. The small ball-shaped attachment appears to be a favorite among many women. Again, choice here is totally individual. Some women prefer a gentle vibrator while others like a heavier, more powerful machine. If the sensation is too strong, use a towel or some clothing between your body and the vibrator to soften the sensations. When Janice found the vibrator stimulation too intense, she would move the vibrator elsewhere around her body and then back to her genitals again after a few moments. "Sex is more physical than I gave it credit for," she ultimately decided.

Some women are hesitant to use a vibrator for fear that they will get "hooked" on it and not be able to have orgasms any other way. First of all, if you haven't been experiencing orgasm at all, using a vibrator surely can do no harm, especially since there is an excellent chance that you'll become orgasmic this way. Secondly, there is no evidence that women who have orgasms with vibrators are unable to have orgasms with other kinds of stimulation. However, stimulation produced by using water or a vibrator is unique, so women who may be orgasmic easily with a vibrator may have to spend more time when other types of touch are used.

A vibrator sometimes stimulates the urethra, which may result in unintentional urination. If this should happen to you, practice the Kegel exercises. Urinate before using the vibrator and put a towel on the bed if it makes you feel more secure. But really, why should we be so concerned over expelling a few drops of urine?

Using a vibrator may be equivalent to using training wheels to learn to ride a bicycle. You get the feeling of what the experience is like and then, if you want to, you can practice without the machine. However, there is no reason to stop using a vibrator, either alone or with a partner, if you enjoy it. Many women have very successfully integrated the vibrator into their sexual relationship with a partner before, during, after, or instead of intercourse. Some men enjoy the sensation of the vibrator on their bodies and genitals too.

If the masturbation is working and you are beginning to feel new and different sexual feelings, you may find this as upsetting as not feeling any sensations at all. Angela found that the more she became interested in sex and enjoyed it, the more guilty she felt. As we feel more, it seems that the old sexual taboos can come back to haunt us. We think we have gotten over the guilt and fears, and then they show up again to plague us once more: Maybe we really will lose consciousness or become a nymphomaniac. Let the fears come. Exaggerate them! What is your worst fantasy? That you'll sleep with every man in town and that your telephone number will be found on the walls of men's rooms? Let your fears take over, follow them to their limit—no matter how absurd they become. Trying to ignore the fears and pretend that they aren't there often requires more energy than giving them full rein. Reality is rarely as bad as your worst fears.

Karen McLellan, who leads pre-orgasmic women's groups in Berkeley, California, talks about a lesson she learned from tai chi: "If something's coming at you (your fears, for example) and you try to force that thing back, then it ultimately gets you. At the very least, all your energy is wasted holding it at bay. So I say, when your bad feelings come in, don't try to force them away. Let them come; and then say, 'Oh, it's just that stuff again. Oh yes, I know you. So long, I'm doing something else now; I'll get to you later.'"

As you masturbate, let the fears come. Try to make them bigger; then smaller. Have fun changing the size and intensity of the fears. Play with them and let them wash over you like waves. Getting to know them well can keep them from seeming so overwhelming, so scary, and prevent them from interfering with your sexual progress.

Some women experience intense feelings when they first begin the masturbation assignments and then suddenly feel nothing during successive efforts. If this happens to you, don't worry—if you could feel the sensations once, you can feel them again. More than likely, the intensity of the initial sensations frightened you and caused you to hold back. Discontinue the masturbation for a few days and then very slowly begin again.

Become familiar with your new sexual feelings. You don't have to discover the whole range in one day or even one week. Move on slowly and push a little bit further ahead each time. It's like going out on a branch for an apple. You can creep out a bit, then move back to where it feels safer, then creep out just a tiny bit more, then back again, and then another tiny move out. Soon you'll feel safe at the beginning of the branch and frightened only when you get out toward the end near the apple. Little by little, with continuous testing, you'll slowly begin to feel safe with the new sensations. You'll learn to trust yourself and the branch. You won't lose control and fall. The branch remains stable and the apple is almost within reach.

Getting close to orgasm can feel like a sneeze that doesn't quite happen. Frequently, reaching these high levels of excitement without release can be as irritating and frustrating as that lost sneeze. The women with whom I work call these levels of excitation "plateaus." All the excitement and sexual tension is there, but they are not yet able to move beyond to orgasm. After a number of sessions that end at this plateau, women can become quite demoralized and discouraged.

The responsibility for overcoming this last barrier to reaching orgasm is primarily yours. Try to push beyond this point by stimulating yourself a few seconds beyond the time when you would ordinarily stop. With each succeeding session, continue the stimulation until you reach a level of slightly higher intensity before stopping. Sometimes the feelings will build and at other times they will diminish. Just at the point you may think that you've lost them forever, they may suddenly return.

If you are stuck at the high plateau level but have not succeeded in going over it to experience the release of orgasm, you're probably expending as much energy fighting the orgasm as you are trying to make it happen. Relax, but don't stop the stimulation. There is one kind of muscular tension that fights the orgasm and another kind that enhances it. If you feel your whole body becoming as tight as a spring, try to relax, but continue to stimulate the genital area. Breathe deeply; imagine the air being breathed in and out of your vagina, rather than your nose or mouth. This helps to ease the anxiety. Change positions to eliminate some of the excess tension. If breathing deeply and regularly doesn't work, maybe you need to hold your breath.

Lydia found that holding her breath helped her get over the plateau stage while Sally needed to breathe deeply. Experiment with several different breathing patterns to see what works for you; for example, some women prefer panting in short rhythmic gasps.

If you are becoming extremely frustrated, get up and take a thirty-second walk; look out the window. One of the women in the group would get up and brush her teeth when she felt stuck. Stopping won't cause you to lose the feelings completely. They'll return when you start to stimulate yourself again.

Building up sexual tension, letting it ebb and then increasing it again, can produce a level of arousal that can be somewhat frightening. Some women fear that the release won't be great enough for the tension that has been built up, or that the release will be too great. How can you be sure that you won't explode or disintegrate if all that tension is unleashed? Intellectually, you may know that you won't, but the intensity of the feelings could make you hold back.

The experience of reaching the plateau and not being able to get over reminds me of a situation I encountered while learning rock climbing. To descend over a steep face, the rock climber must use a rope fastened around his or her backside at one end and attached to a tree or another climber at the other end. This process is called rappelling. A good friend and I were atop a forty-foot sheer face where she was teaching me how to rappel. I turned my back to the edge and took a timid step backward. The objective was to step backward off the ledge and lower myself slowly, using the rope for support. I knew all this intellectually, but I still had to take that last step backward over the edge. I became more and more frightened. I took a few deep breaths. I walked forward and stopped, then stepped slowly backward to the edge of the cliff, unable to step off. I repeated this process a dozen times without going over, despite valid assurances that it was absolutely safe. After the twelfth time, I finally decided in my own head that I would have to force myself to step off the cliff into the abyss. So, I took a deep breath, relaxed my body, and stepped off, feeling totally panicked for one split second as I weightlessly dropped over the edge a tiny distance before the support of the rope securely held me and I began to lower myself down. After that, it became progressively easier each time I had to step off the edge until, after a while, I could rappel with no difficulty whatsoever. The type of determination required to go over the edge of the cliff is similar to that required to have an orgasm. Despite what anyone says, you may still experience that split second of fear. "Will I really fall into nothingness?" you may ask. The only way to convince yourself you'll survive is to relax and let go. Passing through that fear will bring you to the other side. Both the pleasure of the experience and the attainment of the goal are worth the risk.

The turning point for Carmen came when she remembered what Katie had told her. After Katie had experienced her first orgasm, she said to Carmen, "If you *want* it to work, it *does* work. It will happen if you just let go." In order for Judy to have an orgasm, she imagined the whole group saying, "It's OK, Judy." Carol became orgasmic when she decided *not* to stop the pleasurable feelings even though she wasn't expecting to have an orgasm.

Evelyn had an orgasm after deciding she couldn't control other things in her life, especially her financial problems. So she put all her energy into attempting to solve her sexual problem, and she had two orgasms that day!

If old fears and concerns return they can be combated. Cindy borrowed a friend's vibrator. While her children were too busy watching TV to interrupt her, she spent two hours masturbating but had her first orgasm within the first hour.

After it was over, she wondered if she had really had one. She said, "I had this tickling sensation. My body was lifting up and I was trying to get more sensation. I was moving my body around and my nipples became erect. Then came this scared feeling I always have, but I stuck with it and it went away. I held my breath and really felt good, giggly, warm. It was fast. The tickling sensation came, I let go, and felt fine again. I tried breathing and this intensified the feeling. Eventually I continued without the vibrator."

Some women find that they get unstuck if they role-play. When you reach a plateau, move your body around as if you were having an orgasm. Elaborate on the pretend orgasm. Act as if it were very intense. Make lots of sounds and exaggerate the body movements. Sarah did this, and to her surprise a real orgasm followed soon after the simulated one.

Don't give up, but if you feel discouraged and frustrated don't pretend that those feelings don't exist, either. Rather, attempt to get in deeper touch with them. Allow your whole body to feel disheartened. Consider the possibility that you may never allow yourself to take that final leap, because only you can do it for yourself. Janice was very discouraged, and I told her to get in touch with the fact that she might never have an orgasm. I told her to go home and really think about that possibility. This made her furious. She said, "Why should I get in touch with never having an orgasm? I've been in touch with that for thirty years. I'm not going to think about that. I'm going to have it if it kills me!" And she did—the very next day.

Don't forget about experimenting with the expression of other feelings, too, if you have a tendency to keep everything, including sexual feelings, safely locked inside. Holding emotions inside requires a tremendous amount of energy, energy that could be better used in being creative, productive, feeling intimate and sexual. Experiment for a week or two. Allow your feelings to "hang out" for that length of time by expressing them as soon as you are aware of them. If you tend to cover things over with a smile, it may be especially important to practice sharing your feelings. Ellen had a fight with her husband. It was the first time she had expressed her anger in a long time. When she did the exercises that night, she had her first orgasm. She said it measured 10 on the Richter scale.

In general, however, first orgasms are not very intense. They take a long time to achieve and may be barely noticeable. Sometimes women are disappointed after all the work and effort. The lack of intensity in the beginning frequently results from the amount of energy invested in fighting the orgasm. As you experience more orgasms and become less afraid and anxious, the orgasms can become more powerful. However, some women prefer mild orgasms. Kelly had mild orgasms and liked them exactly as they were.

After experiencing the first orgasm, many women become afraid that they won't be able to have another one. Frequently, they repeat the exercises immediately to see if it happens again. After one orgasm, Laurie kept masturbating over and over again to make sure it was really true. Sherry re-created the exact scene to ensure that the orgasm would be repeated. Women are often afraid that the newfound skill will disappear unless they follow the magical method that caused it to occur the first time. It takes a while before you can be comfortable and assured that orgasm will occur. Most of the time it will. Occasionally it won't, so don't worry, it's not lost. You may have to relax a bit more, or be more in the mood.

Sometimes the orgasm doesn't come because you're trying to force it to happen. It seems that when the pressure is turned on, the orgasm is turned off. Laurie found it helped to just enjoy the feelings without having to reach an orgasm. Inevitably, when she could relax and feel good with no goal in mind, the orgasm would occur.

Sexual sensations ebb and flow. You may feel turned on, and then lose the feeling. There is no need to struggle for the lost sensation as another one will develop soon if you relax. Sexual feelings are like waves in the ocean. There is no need to break your neck to catch a particular wave when you can relax and wait for another one. There are an infinite number of waves in the sea, and an infinite number of orgasms.

First, learn to be comfortable about having orgasms on your own. Then you can try to integrate them into your lovemaking with your partner—if you want to. Sherry found that she really needed to experience orgasm by herself before she was ready to share it with her partner. Nina, on the other hand, was orgasmic with her husband almost immediately after she had one by herself. Every woman is different. Check and see what is comfortable for you.

Leslie's husband was upset because he said sex wasn't any better for him even though she had become orgasmic. This put her under pressure to have her orgasms for his pleasure and not for herself. She finally got up the nerve to set him straight. She had waited forty-eight years to be orgasmic and now he could wait to share them.

Once you are experiencing orgasms with masturbation, you may find sex with your partner disappointing. This is not uncommon. Polly became comfortable with masturbation, and enjoyed the orgasms which resulted, but she felt frustrated by lovemaking with her partner because she could not attain the same release. Soon, however, when the novelty of masturbation wore off, Polly renewed her interest in partner sex again. Janice was just the opposite. Before she entered the group she avoided sex whenever possible, but once she began having orgasms with masturbation, her opinion toward sex changed. She wasn't having orgasms with her partner yet, but she was enjoying sex; her whole attitude was more positive.

Whether or not you are orgasmic with your partner, there is no reason to stop masturbating. Instead of looking at self-stimulation from an antiquated perspective—as a substitute for the "real thing"—why not view it as one of many alternative forms of sexual expression—provided by nature for a party of one.

9: Elaborating on What You've Learned

If you have recently learned to masturbate or even if you have been orgasmic with masturbation through most of your life, you may not find yourself totally at ease with the experience. In my first pre-orgasmic women's group, I set out to advocate masturbation to other women even though I was not as yet totally accepting of the idea myself. However, through the course of my work, this feeling changed. My experience demonstrates that it is possible to learn about one's sexuality through self-stimulation without first being completely at ease with the idea. Comfort with masturbation may only come with time and positive experience.

One way to begin exploring self-stimulation further is by making it a new and different experience. Experiment by doing something you've never tried before. Carol stroked her body with feathers, silk, leather, and other textured materials before and during masturbation.

Many women have a tendency to remain dissatisfied. In the therapy program, some women argued that orgasms with masturbation were not "real" or worthwhile. Women who are already orgasmic may grumble because they are not *multi*-orgasmic. Others who are multiorgasmic may complain that their orgasms aren't intense enough. Those who have to fantasize to achieve orgasm may label themselves abnormal. Those who don't fantasize may feel that they are missing out. One way or another, you can find ways to negate your experiences if you want to.

If you would like to intensify your orgasmic response or experience multiple orgasms, there are techniques that might enable you to do so. You can experiment with these and see if you like the results, or if you prefer your original pattern.

The most effective way to intensify an orgasm is by prolonging the pleasurable experience preceding it through a process called "teasing." First, build genital tension and maintain it at a peak but don't let yourself get excited enough to reach orgasm. Stimulate yourself a bit, enough to get closer but not too close to orgasm, and then change the site of stimulation to an area that is less sensitive. Or use a lighter, more delicate, teasing touch. Feel the level of arousal rise and drop, then hang suspended. Take your time, enjoy the feelings. Keep up the teasing for a while before intensifying the stimulation sufficiently to trigger the orgasm. Teasing allows for a greater buildup of sexual tension, and the more tension that is built up, the greater the orgasmic release.

Instead of fighting the pleasure, ride it like a wave—submerged and synchronized. If you relax and flow with the feelings, a more intense orgasm should result. *Consciously* relax. Use some deep breathing techniques.[1] (For example, close your eyes and imagine that there is a screen directly in front of your eyes. Focus on the screen and let any images that appear pass through or bounce off the screen. Meanwhile breathe in deeply through your mouth. Then close your mouth and as you exhale, imagine you are actually breathing the air out through your vagina.) Prolonging the feelings and flowing freely with them is the key to a more intense response.

Miscalculation, however, can result in a disappointing experience. Betty employed the teasing technique, but when she built up the tension for the third time, she misjudged her level of arousal and accidentally stimulated herself to orgasm. Not being prepared for it, she experienced almost no satisfaction or release.

Another way to intensify orgasm is through exaggeration. Many women keep their bodies totally passive while stimulating the genital area. This may create a split between the active sexual self and the passive, resisting self. To reduce this split, stimulate other erotically sensitive areas in addition to your genitals. Getting your whole body into the sexually active state can enhance the experience. Ellen exaggerated everything. She moved her body more, made more sounds, breathed more deeply, and created more muscle tension. The result met her expectations—an intensified orgasm and a greater sense of release and accompanying relaxation.

Making sounds can be difficult for men as well as women. It is almost as if in the heat of passion we are still attempting to look dignified. Constantly and painfully aware of how others may be viewing us, we remain carefully quiet. Withholding noises during sex can have a stifling effect on orgasm. You may not naturally feel like making sounds, and that is fine, but if you are carefully guarding against vocalizing, you are not as free to let go completely. Sally's orgasms really began to change when she felt the freedom to express outwardly what she felt inwardly both in terms of sounds and body movements.

If you would like to experience multiple orgasms or a slightly different type of orgasmic pattern, you might want to try a vibrator/massager. Vibrators provide a consistent intensity that cannot be duplicated manually. As a result, the stimulation provided by a vibrator may be sufficient to bring you to orgasm one or more times with minimal effort.

Orgasms with vibrators may differ in some respects from those produced by other kinds of stimulation. The buildup with a vibrator may be very brief; in fact, some women find it too brief to achieve the desired release. Other women like the vibrator precisely because it takes so little time and energy. Women who say that an orgasm with a vibrator feels like an electrical charge coursing through their bodies are those who prefer the slower, more gradual buildup and release provided by manual stimulation.

Vibrators can be enjoyed as additions to solo or shared sexual experiences. However, some women who object to the technological computer-instant-freeze-dried orientation of society may classify vibrators with frozen TV dinners, tape-recorded answering services, and microwave ovens. These women generally prefer a return to the more natural, slower, less complicated human functions. Thus, philosophically, they might find a vibrator unappealing.

Other women express the fear that they will turn into "vibrator junkies" and never be satisfied sexually by any other method of stimulation. To date, this has not generally been a problem. However, some women do tend to get spoiled by the rapidity with which they experience orgasm with a vibrator and may become discouraged with the slower process of having orgasms with manual stimulation. Switching from a vibrator to manual stimulation may mean investing more time in masturbation, but you can probably make the switch if you have an interest in doing so. Harriet experienced her first orgasm with a vibrator and continued to use it both alone and with her partner. After six months she decided to try reaching orgasm manually; it was like learning to have an orgasm again for the first time. It took her several days of doing the exercises before, after forty minutes of manual stimulation, she finally had her first orgasm without a vibrator. She was elated and vowed to use manual stimulation along with the vibrator from then on.

One way that might make the transition from vibrator to manual stimulation easier is to use the vibrator until you experience a high level of arousal and then switch to manual stimulation. The following time, discontinue use of the vibrator at a slightly lower level of arousal. Continue this process until you find that you are able to begin the self-stimulation without use of the vibrator.

Various vibrator substitutes have been reported by women in the groups. And, of course, the sensations produced by the running water technique are similar to those produced by a vibrator. A statement by Phillis Lyon and Del Martin in *Lesbian Woman* aptly makes the distinction between the physiological and psychological aspects of orgasm. "As Masters and Johnson so well argued, an orgasm is an orgasm, no matter how it is achieved the body goes through the same physiological pattern, whether orgasm comes through a loved one or a vibrating washing machine. The 'quality' of the orgasm differs—not within the body, but within the head. There is, after all, a great deal of difference psychologically between your lover and your washing machine."[2] However, this does not mean that you can't enjoy them both. The only way to find out is to try it.

In order to explore the range of your sexual response and to begin training yourself to experience orgasms with lovemaking, it may be necessary for you to try a variety of positions and techniques during masturbation that resemble those used with a partner. Many women use only one method to masturbate and this is the way they have learned to respond orgasmically. Often, this approach is not adaptable to partner sex, and it may be necessary to learn new techniques that are easier to use with your partner. Learning to respond in other ways requires a bit of experimentation.

Explore different positions. If you've been lying on your back, bring your knees up to your chest. Try lying on your stomach or in a kneeling position as if there were a partner beneath you. Gradually change the focal point and type of self-stimulation so that it approaches techniques used by a partner. Sensitize your clitoral area to the subtler stimulation resulting from intercourse by lightly stroking this area for twenty minutes a day over a period of about two weeks.

In preparation for orgasm with a partner, practice increasing the sensitivity of the vagina by inserting your fingers or other phallic-shaped objects that will not splinter, cut, or in other ways injure the tissues. Kinsey found that 20 percent of the masturbating females reported using vaginal insertions some of the time to provide vaginal stimulation while the clitoral area was simultaneously stimulated manually or mechanically.[3] Although terribly embarrassed, Diane finally disclosed to the group that she had been masturbating by moving a perfume bottle in and out of her vagina. She found this experience very stimulating, and with the aid of fantasy, one which closely resembled the sensation of intercourse. However, she began to notice a vague burning sensation in her vagina and thought it best to discontinue using the bottle. Since that time she has continued to use other, safer dildoes to enhance her masturbation.

Compare the sensations you experience with a partner to those you feel when you stimulate yourself while alone. Can you begin to identify when you are turning off or discern what is lacking? Remember that while the experience of orgasm with masturbation may be psychologically different from an orgasmic experience with your partner, physiologically it is the same. However, some attitudes or a lack of skill may be preventing you from utilizing the common elements of the two experiences and transferring the orgasm from masturbation to sex with your partner.

10: Rethinking Sexual Goals

Myths and misinformation are major obstacles to enjoying sex fully and becoming orgasmic with a partner. The following myths have been mentioned earlier in the book, but will be repeated here because they often play a significant role in circumscribing our sexual activities and shaping our notions of what is considered "normal" sexual behavior.

The first myth, and the one that is the most difficult to dispel, is that the so-called "vaginal orgasm" is somehow superior. I hope the information in this book and others has finally put an end to that myth.[1] A woman who needs more clitoral stimulation than that indirectly provided by the thrusting of the penis to achieve orgasm is no more abnormal than a man who requires very rapid thrusting to achieve his climax.

Recent research indicates that most women, although not all, require some amount of direct clitoral stimulation, just as most men require some direct penile stimulation, in order to reach orgasm. About one quarter of the women who completed the group therapy program could achieve orgasm through intercourse alone, at least occasionally, while two thirds were able to achieve orgasm if clitoral stimulation accompanied intercourse. These results are similar to a study carried out by *Forum* magazine where only one fifth of the self-selected respondents found penile-vaginal thrusting sufficient to achieve orgasm while three fifths of the sample needed a combination of clitoral and vaginal stimulation and one fifth required clitoral stimulation alone.[2]

A friend of mine was involved with a woman he liked very much but was disturbed because she didn't reach orgasm. Finally he asked her if she could have orgasms by herself if she masturbated. She was taken aback by the question but finally admitted that she could. He asked her to touch herself the same way she did when she was by herself, while they had intercourse. It took quite a while the first time, but finally she did have an orgasm. It was her first with a partner. She was so delighted that her pleasure overcame her embarrassment.

Some women can have orgasms solely through intercourse with certain men and not others. Relationship problems aside, this may occur because of a man's particular rhythm of thrusting or the shape of his pubic bone which allows for more or less direct clitoral stimulation. Is this woman abnormal with one partner and normal with the other? Should she end the relationship with a man she loves simply because in order for her to experience orgasm, their lovemaking must include other modes of stimulation in addition to intercourse? No. It's absurd that so much emphasis is placed on the manner in which an orgasm is attained rather than the enjoyment two people derive from their lovemaking. Nina could have orgasms with intercourse plus clitoral stimulation, but wouldn't let herself accept them as valid. She kept believing the myth that it wasn't the *right* way.

Some women say that orgasms achieved through vaginal thrusting are "different" or "more satisfying." If you don't have orgasms this way, you may assume this is true and that you are missing something. Having a penis contained within the vagina may enhance sexual pleasure before and during orgasm, but this doesn't preclude the addition of direct clitoral stimulation.

Why not do away with the myth that there are better and worse ways of having an orgasm? Instead, acknowledge that having orgasms through intercourse without additional stimulation may not be possible given your unique physiological makeup or the anatomic fit with your partner.

If someone came to you desiring to learn to fly but refusing to use any props to help her, you would be likely to think her absurd; she *might* succeed, but it would be highly improbable. If, however, she would use a glider or some paraphernalia designed specifically to assist in flying, she would probably succeed. Apply this analogy to attaining orgasm. You might succeed without clitoral stimulation, but with it you have a much better chance. The pleasure of the orgasm is the same either way—so why make things difficult for yourself?

The second myth is that sex and intercourse are synonymous; that all sexual encounters must include or culminate in intercourse and orgasm must occur during intercourse; that nothing else is considered "normal." However, intercourse is only one of a number of ways to give and receive sexual pleasure. Sexual relationships and sexual feelings extend far beyond the act of intercourse. To make intercourse the goal of sex does a grave disservice to many enjoyable ways of touching. It somehow implies that other sexual activities don't count or aren't important.

The term *sex* includes anything that turns you on and gives you sexual pleasure. It doesn't have to include a partner, but it can. It doesn't have to include orgasm, but that's a possibility. It doesn't even have to include any genital touching—it could just consist of fantasy. The feelings can last for hours or pass in a flash. You can write your own scripts for each sexual experience and each one may be different. But most important, it doesn't *have* to end in intercourse. Other modes of sexual stimulation can comprise a complete sexual experience or intercourse can be enjoyable as foreplay or afterplay.

Another overrated myth is the superiority of the simultaneous orgasm. Both people "should" climax together in one glorious mind-bending explosion. Striving for a simultaneous orgasm can require considerable concentration on what your lover is experiencing and less concentration on and enjoyment of your own experience. Achieving a simultaneous orgasm can require a lot of carefully controlled strategy as opposed to free abandon. "Is he almost there? How fast is he breathing? He's almost there and I'm not; what'll I do?" These thoughts alone can block an individual orgasm, much less a simultaneous one. You may find it more enjoyable for you and your partner to experience consecutive orgasms; in this way you can concentrate totally on your own sexual buildup and release and then concentrate totally on pleasuring your partner and experiencing your partner's excitement and release and vice versa. If you experience simultaneous orgasm, fine; that can be one kind of experience, but not necessarily one to strive for each time. Kelly prefers having consecutive orgasms because then she can relate more to her partner. She said that if they have orgasms at the same time, they both feel more isolated because they are so involved in their own pleasure. Ann said she prefers to have her orgasm first. Then she can better enjoy pleasuring her lover because she feels satisfied, and close to him. Other women like their partners to climax first because then they feel that they can finally relax and become immersed in the sexual sensations. Finding patterns that fit for you with as much or as little variation as you desire is essential.

Another important myth to dispel is the belief that the male must be aggressive and the female passive; that it is unfeminine to be sexually assertive and unmasculine to remain passive sexually. If we accept this belief, we prevent the woman from being innovative and expressing her needs and desires and we prohibit the man from being able to relax and enjoy being pleasured.

Opening up the relationship to sexual changes initiated by you can pave the way for vast improvements. Since many of us have been taught that we should not enjoy sex or be sexually aggressive, we take a very passive role in lovemaking, expecting our partners to initiate while we remain passively receptive. Sex becomes a dance where the male leads and the female follows. The dance may become routine, since the male partner knows only a limited number of steps. Dancing (and sex) could be twice as interesting if the female would also initiate and add steps of her own. Most men enjoy the opportunity of having a partner assume some responsibility for sexual initiation and innovation.[3] It takes some of the burden off them. According to Moulton, "The woman who feels free to be physically active in lovemaking usually makes a more exciting partner than one who never expresses her own erotic preferences or who takes no initiative, feeling that her role is merely to follow and please the man. This may be gratifying to some men initially, but it is apt to become stereotyped and lifeless to both partners."[4]

Being able to assert yourself is essential because no one can read your mind. You are going to have to take the initiative in your sexual relationship to make certain that your needs are met. It means assuming more responsibility for yourself. By doing so, you gain a sense of autonomy that allows you to have sex if you want to, or refuse it if you're not in the mood. Some women get into the bind of resisting sex simply because their partner initiates it. They begin to feel that sex is something that is "done" to them, an activity in which they can make no choices. However, once you feel the freedom to initiate sex and take part in directing it, it can be as enjoyable for you as it is for your partner. Sherry used to freeze up when her husband made sexual advances toward her. But now she says, "I realize that I can be in control and do not have to be a spectator watching what he does to me. I stop and think for a moment, 'Do *I* want sex?' If the answer is no I tell him, and if the answer is yes I can leap in and enjoy it." Laurie uses the vibrator during intercourse and really enjoys the fabulous feelings she didn't have before. She says, "Now I'm a willing partner and equal in initiating sex. Now I don't feel like pushing him away when he becomes amorous because I have the freedom to say, 'No, I'm tired and let's try it tomorrow,' because now I'm being honest."

Frequently your sexual desire or lack of it will coincide with that of your partner, but even if it doesn't, masturbation provides each partner the freedom to express their individual sexual needs even when the other person is not in the mood to participate. Surprisingly enough, most couples' frequency of sexual contact rises rather than declines once both partners feel that they have the freedom to refuse sex if they choose to do so.

And that leads me to the last myth, the notion that sex "should" come naturally—that is, we should intuitively and automatically know what our partner likes and wants at a specific moment and our partner should be able to mind-read our desires. Perhaps the most important contribution to a satisfying sexual relationship is the ability to communicate with a partner. Each of us is unique and the only way our partner can know what we want is if we communicate. We need to develop our own individual styles, and redefine sexuality so that it fits each of us individually. If we like one technique or position we can engage in it and if not, we can forget it. The fact that we like or don't like a specific activity is reason enough for our doing or not doing it. And there is always the possibility that the activities we reject today may be acceptable tomorrow.

However, likes and dislikes often vary between sexual partners and compromises have to be made. For example, if your partner hates spinach and you really like it, there is no reason why you would have to give up spinach altogether. Either you'll prepare spinach less frequently or else you'll provide carrots for your partner and spinach for yourself. Likewise with sex. A couple can use certain positions occasionally, if they are enjoyable only for one person, while employing additional positions—some that are your favorites, some that are your partner's, and especially those that you enjoy equally. If you both are getting what you want, there is less likely to be resentment and conflict over sexual activities.

Myths change slowly. You may find yourself intellectually thinking that some of these myths make little sense as rigid rules for behavior while emotionally continuing to respond in accordance with them. Changing basic beliefs takes time; they don't automatically vanish just because you confront them. Rather, positive personal experience is the most effective means of changing beliefs. For example, let's say that you had always been told, and therefore believed, that all frozen orange juice tasted the same, so you always bought the most inexpensive brand. Then you visited a friend for breakfast and the orange juice tasted fresh. When you inquired about it, she told you that it was a different brand of frozen juice from the one you usually bought. You might then not only change brands of orange juice, but alter your belief that all frozen orange juice tastes alike. Similarly with sex: Through personal experience, you can learn to identify your own needs, wants, and patterns of response. I am not issuing a blanket statement that sex in all forms is marvelous and that anything "should" go. Such a statement is as coercive as the religious doctrines that dictate that sex is permissible only for the purposes of procreation. To be sure, sex is fun, but each of us has a different idea of what "fun" means. Some of us may ride motorcycles for enjoyment while others play bridge, and there is plenty of room for these individual preferences. We have the right to choose what forms of sex are enjoyable for us. But let us look to our own commonsense response and not the "shoulds" of others to make our decisions. Let us respect the rights and needs of others while we explore our own needs and preferences, slowly and carefully, trying only the things that feel right to try at a particular time. In this way, we can escape the chains of myth and social stereotype and experience the freedom of expressing our authentic selves.

11: Partners

Once you are orgasmic through self-stimulation, the next step is sharing your sexuality—integrating the process into a sexual relationship with a partner. Whatever the nature of your partner relationship, you may have to confront some significant issues in order to make the changes that will enable you to be orgasmic with your partner.

Before you even begin to talk to your partner about altering your sexual relationship, it is natural for you to wonder what response you'll get. Why should your partner want to make changes? If sex has not been satisfying for you and you've talked about it with your partner, your partner probably isn't totally satisfied either. Even if you've been faking orgasms and your partner is unaware of your dissatisfaction, there are still many benefits to making changes in your sexual routine—benefits for both of you.

Any couple's sex life can get into a rut after a period of time. Making alterations can sometimes provide a refreshing change. Just talking about sex and thinking about it at various times during the day can enhance your relationship.

Prolonging the lovemaking, making it a voluptuous meal rather than a quick snack, can replace humdrum sex with real excitement. Spending the time enjoying the scenery along the way rather than doggedly focusing on the destination can result in a much more relaxing and sensuous experience. And the longer and more enjoyable the whole experience is, the more likely it is to include orgasm.

Self-stimulation has taught you what arouses you and you now know some things that you can teach your partner which will add to the lovemaking experience. Teaching your partner what excites you sexually can relieve performance pressure. Once a male partner is comfortable with manual and other techniques, he will not need to maintain an erection for an extended period of time, or get an erection at all, for you to attain orgasm.

Sex, although only one aspect of a relationship, is an important aspect. Being close and communicating about sex can bring a deeper level of communication in all aspects of the relationship. Pleasing each other in bed can spread to pleasing each other in areas outside the bedroom. Open sexual communication can mean the difference between sexual frustration and satisfaction.

The end results can be delightful—but getting to the end is not simple. As a matter of fact, the most difficult part often occurs in making the first move. How to bring up the subject of sex and how to discuss it openly presents great obstacles to many women. You may find yourself wanting to quit even before you've begun.

You may hesitate to talk to your partner for reasons that go deeper than a mere reluctance to talk openly about sex. You may be angry at your partner for things that you haven't expressed openly. Some women feel powerless in their relationship. They may feel that the only time they can say no is in bed. If you say no or argue about what is really bothering you, you might fear that you will stir up a fight or even ultimately lose your partner. So maybe you take out your resentments by withholding sex. Some women acquiesce to sex, but get even with their partners by not having orgasms. We're all unfortunately too familiar with the martyred wife: "I'll go along with sex, but I'll be so frustrated and miserable that you'll be sorry." Your partner may end up feeling lousy, but you will, too. Meanwhile, your partner is unaware of what *really* is bothering you. For all too long, sex has been the battleground for other issues. If you're fighting on the wrong front, you can't possibly win. Maybe you could win, though, if you could argue about what *truly* bothers you, leaving your sexual feelings for your partner uncontaminated by other negative feelings.

Again, fears may get in the way. Deep down, you may fear that you really aren't sexual and that trying to change your orgasmic situation might only confirm this fear.

Some women find it difficult to ask because they fear being turned down. Jenny can't ask for anything until she is desperately in need. Then, if her request is refused, she feels devastated. She and other women like her, who have had no practice at making requests when the stakes are low, never learn to cope with the reactions that occur when they finally do make a request and it is refused.

Also common is the fear of being engulfed if you let go and have an orgasm with your partner. You've learned to trust yourself and your own self-stimulation, but giving that power and control to a partner can be disquieting. You can't give up control unless you feel you have some. Therefore, gaining more control is a task that precedes learning to give it up. Control can be gained by telling your partner what you want. By practicing the yes's and no's described in Chapter 4 you can be convinced that you can stop sex or say no to it anytime you want to. Then, when you feel that you have more control over your sexual decisions, you may find that you feel secure enough to allow yourself to relax and let go.

Sherry was afraid to let her orgasmic feelings engulf her with her husband—even though she could enjoy those feelings when alone. She would find herself involuntarily holding back during partner lovemaking. With time and practice, however, she slowly learned to trust herself and her responses with her partner as well.

You may be afraid you'll hurt your partner's feelings and so you protect him by not doing anything about your lack of orgasmic response. You may be afraid of hurting his ego or threatening him. Is your partner really that fragile? Do you have to remain the pure little girl for him to feel like the potent man? If you become more responsive, will he feel inferior as a man? There is no way to second-guess his reaction for sure, but you may be wasting years of sexual enjoyment for yourself while needlessly protecting him. It may be better to take a chance and attempt to make some changes. Keep in mind that making changes is not always easy, nor does it always happen without any unpleasant, guilty, or uncertain feelings. There is risk involved, but generally far less a risk than you might imagine.

The status quo might be unhappy, but at least you're familiar with it, and it feels safe. Rocking the boat by trying to modify your sex life might produce a type of unhappiness for which you are unprepared. What happens if it fails? Then what? Or worse still, what happens if he stops loving you, or if he leaves you because of your attempts to make sex better for yourself? Granted, making changes in a relationship is difficult and potentially disruptive, but doing nothing and remaining dissatisfied is usually far worse. If you do take the risk and attempt to make the alterations you desire, you'll probably discover that your fears were exaggerated.

Negative male reactions to changing sexual behavior can occur, especially at the beginning. Change may not always be well received by your partner; he may not love them immediately. He may even be upset. Some men are threatened by women masturbating and fear that they might be replaced by masturbation. Many men feel astounded that you would want to masturbate when they are there to meet your sexual needs. Initially masturbation may also be as unacceptable to him as it was to you. Both men and women have been brought up in the same culture and have been indoctrinated with similar feelings about self-stimulation.

If your partner objects to your suggestions initially, he will probably mellow with time, assuming that you care for him and that you're sincerely interested in making your sexual relationship better. You may want to let him know that many men react this way at first. It may help him to better understand and accept his response. Ann's husband felt better after she told him that the partners of other women in the group were threatened, too.

Some men feel inadequate if you open the subject of sex— especially if they weren't previously aware that there was a problem. Until you explain the difficulty he may feel that your lack of orgasmic response is his fault. Even if your partner is aware that you have trouble reaching orgasm, he may feel that his sexual technique is deficient or that he is inadequate as a lover, especially if he accepts the myth that he "should" be the authority on sex rather than looking to you for more information and direction.

Both Angela's and Gloria's husbands were very threatened the first week of the group. Gloria's husband ejaculated prematurely several times and Angela's husband was unable to get an erection on two occasions. Within a week both problems had passed, but Angela's husband threatened to divorce her if his problem were to continue and she refused to quit the group. It is interesting to note that Angela never threatened to divorce *him* if her problem continued.

Women are often willing to assume the role of patient, understanding, forgiving sexual companion. How ludicrous it would appear if roles were reversed and women usually had their orgasms first, rolled off their partners, and went to sleep. If the man protested, the woman could explain that she was too tired to go on and apologize. I wonder how many men would acquiesce and say, "It's OK, dear, it doesn't matter."

The group experiences indicate, however, that most partners' reactions are positive and supportive, if not initially, then after a very short period of time. Some men are concerned that they won't be able to change enough to meet the needs of their partners. Harriet's husband was so desperately eager to please her that he was very worried about his ability to make the changes Harriet wanted.

Most men are very appreciative when they are finally given information they can apply to lovemaking. Frequently, these men have tried everything and don't know what else to do to improve the situation. Receiving assistance from a partner relieves them of the responsibility for finding a solution. Most men will cooperate once they understand how important the issue of your sex life is to you.

If you and your partner don't generally talk very openly about sex, inserting the topic into general conversation can be tricky. Many couples are stuck in neutral silence: "I won't say anything if you don't, and we'll both pretend there is no problem, that nothing is wrong." But ignoring a problem can ensure that no solution will ever be found, especially if it hasn't worked itself out by now.

Guard against playing "blackmail," that is, when one person brings up a sensitive and touchy issue, the partner retaliates in kind. ("If you want to talk about sex, I want to talk about your mother.") These pacts can destroy closeness and intimacy in a relationship and preclude deeper understanding and change. You want your partner to hear, but you don't want to make him angry, defensive, or hurt. It is difficult to ensure that none of these negative reactions will occur. An initial negative reaction may be inevitable, but much of the reaction depends on the way you present the issue. You can use it as a sledgehammer—"You had better do this or else"—or as a possibility for growth—"There are some things we could change that might make sex more enjoyable for both of us." You can blame your partner—"It's all your fault that our sex life is so lousy, so *you* do something about it." Or you can open up and share your feelings—"Sex hasn't been the best it could be for me, but if you would work on it with me I think there are some things we could do together that might make it better." Take the time to state your personal feelings and fears. Making accusations rarely brings about the desired results. You might want to explain that it is not his fault, but that you have been unaware of how to change the situation; now that you have some idea, you'd like his help.

Sarah had been faking orgasms but finally decided to broach the issue with her partner. She told him, "I'm having trouble reaching orgasm [to say the least—she'd never had an orgasm with a partner], but if you'll give me three hours of your time, we can work on it." She gave him numerous directions during the time that they set aside; they stopped to rest for a while when things did not go well. But after stopping and taking the pressure off, Sarah got closer to having an orgasm than she ever had before, and these first three hours of experimentation remain a memorable experience for them both. Clearly, your initial approach can greatly influence the outcome.

Talking about sex when you have been faking orgasm presents a special difficulty. One woman warned the others not to tell their husbands that they had been faking. She had faked for two years before marriage and two years after. Then, in the heat of an argument, she had told her partner the truth. As a result, their relationship had been going steadily downhill ever since. However, the negative response from her husband may very well have been a reaction to her using the confession of her faking as a weapon in their fight. In my experience, most women who have told their partners in a less emotionally charged atmosphere have met with a more positive response. Nina was finally honest with her partner and to her surprise found that he was very willing to participate in couple's counseling, even though before she had told him, she was sure he would never agree.

You might tell your partner that you are not sure you are having orgasms, or that you would like to try to make them better after reading this book. Carmen used to fake consistently. When she entered the group she told her partner she was going to a class in sexuality; she is now orgasmic but never told him that she once wasn't. In general, follow your intuition and move only as quickly as you feel is prudent in your situation.

Even if your partner is a bit resistant or threatened at first, a loving attitude that takes his uneasiness into account can enable him slowly to feel more secure and more willing to participate. If your partner's initial response is negative, your tendency may be to drop the subject and return to the status quo, even if it's unsatisfactory. However, persistence can bring positive results. Pam was orgasmic with masturbation but never with a partner. She decided that her sexuality was very important and that she wanted to spend time and energy working on it. She presented the idea to her partner, who responded very negatively. He informed her that if she wanted to work on her sexuality, she could do it elsewhere without his participation. Instead of giving up, Pam reiterated that it was important to her and suggested that perhaps he could agree to do just a few things. Finally, he reluctantly agreed to do the assignments. Pam moved slowly and didn't let his lack of enthusiasm get her down. Pam's partner fulfilled each assignment grudgingly, but nonetheless, their sex life improved. They began having sex more frequently, and both felt more sensual and excited than ever before.

Perhaps a good way for you to enlist your partner's cooperation would be to share this book with him. If he will read it, he might better understand the framework for your ideas. In our groups the women are given some written material to read at home. Angela casually left the pamphlets lying around in hopes her husband would notice them. Unfortunately, he never took the hint, or if he did read the material, he never mentioned it. It might be a good idea to be more direct and let your partner know that you want him to read this information.

Discussing sex can lead to closer, deeper feelings, even if it entails some disagreement. At the Medical Center in San Francisco, the Human Sexuality Program periodically presents a two-session sexuality-education program. The first week is devoted to discussion of female sexuality and the second to male sexuality. When couples return the second week after completing the first session, they typically are enthusiastic because they have gone home and talked about sex in a way they never had before. Most of the women report that the sexual experience they had after the talk was one of the best they could remember. A few women have reported that a fight followed the discussion—in some cases a major fight—but that within a day or two they, too, had a close, warm lovemaking session that stood out in their memories.

Talking about sex intimately, openly, and honestly results in being able to talk about other issues more directly. Sex is one of the most personal and difficult areas to discuss. However, once progress has been made in this area, it seems that more honest, open communication takes place in less emotionally charged areas as well.

If you can broach the topic of your sexual relationship with your partner, you have made the first very important step toward improving it. This giant step counts for a lot, even if you have to take a small step backward later. Your partner may need some time to adjust to the idea of relating in a new way sexually. Men have fears and can be uptight about sex, too. For example, some men don't like to touch a woman's genitals; many feel it is morally wrong to stimulate the clitoris. Men may have hangups about nudity or may respond negatively toward a woman who is at all sexually assertive. Harriet's husband was extremely puritanical, but Harriet managed to make some changes in their sex life, by proceeding slowly.

Remember, if you do make some changes in yourself and your approach to sex, your partner will have to interact differently with you, because you will be different. Some women feel that their partners are hopeless and couldn't possibly alter their attitudes toward sex. You may be amazed at the results when you try—not to revise your partner's ideas, but to change *your* role in the sexual relationship. He may not support you at first, but he may respond to the actual sexual experience positively. For change to occur, it is not necessary that your partner take charge; what is necessary is that *you* do some things differently and that he go along with your attempts.

I have given many words of warning and ways to prevent potential difficulties that might deter you from making the changes you desire. But many partners respond optimistically and favorably from the outset. Most lovers care enough about their partners to try almost anything that will increase their mates' happiness. Rather than being an obstacle, your partner could provide support and love, enabling the two of you to transform the exploration of your orgasmic response into an enjoyable game.

Don't expect instantaneous results. Change takes time. Begin by experimenting. The next chapter contains some exercises you can work on with your partner. Allow yourself to relax and enjoy doing them. They have worked for many couples, and with the right approach, they may be helpful for you, too.

12: Partner Exercises

As with the masturbation program, becoming orgasmic with a partner necessitates making the time to practice. This can be a somewhat daunting task, because now two people will have to create blocks of time and synchronize their schedules.

Most couples procrastinate and avoid interacting sexually if their sex life has been less than satisfactory. But if you don't spend time together, things most assuredly will not change. Remember the negative cycle that results from unsatisfying sex. The more negative experiences, the more both people will anticipate a negative experience. This expectation in itself can create enough anxiety and resentment to preclude positive results. Fortunately, positive reinforcement can reverse this process. The more successful experiences you have, the more you will expect a successful outcome, and you can relax, thereby facilitating positive results. Thus, pleasurable experiences are extremely important from the very beginning. Making sure that the time set aside will be relaxing and fairly free from intrusions is absolutely necessary. Moving slowly, going only as far as feels comfortable, and making sure the experience is enjoyable are essential. Keeping communication open about reactions before, during, and after is also critical to paving the way for successful and satisfying lovemaking.

As you begin to experiment, it might be helpful to try to reserve judgment about the exercises. Unless something really offends you, try it a few times, and then decide whether you like it and want to continue using it as one of your options, or if you want to discontinue it temporarily and possibly forever. Remember, all decisions apply only to the present—you can choose to disregard some exercise now, while remaining free to change your mind in the future. If something is making you uncomfortable, be sure to let your partner know. If you don't make yourself clear, your partner may interpret a negative response as a rejection of him rather than of the activity. Adding a positive "Maybe if you tried this" or "Doing it this way might be better," rather than a categorical "Stop" or "Don't do that," is far more instructive and more likely to receive a supportive response.

Since enjoyable sex entails much more than reaching orgasm, it's important to find out exactly what you *are* feeling during sex with a partner, so that you can begin to isolate problem areas. The best way to do this is to forget totally about orgasms for the moment. Treat this as another fact-finding mission and your only assignment is to relax and enjoy the scenery. Concentrate on the sensual feelings. We sometimes put so much emphasis on the goal, orgasm, that we lose track of what we are actually feeling during the sensual experience. Dr. Harvey Caplan, a colleague of mine, tells a story that illustrates the point beautifully. When he was sixteen and just beginning to date and drive, he couldn't wait to park and neck with his current girlfriend. When they stopped driving and began kissing, his mind wasn't on the kissing but on how he could touch her breast. Finally, when he succeeded in that conquest, he couldn't enjoy the feel of her breast because he was already concerned with how he could unfasten her bra. And on and on. He was so busy thinking ahead that he never fully appreciated the feelings of the moment. Many of us still find ourselves in that position today—so concerned about the future, or what's going to happen next, that we don't experience the present.

The first partner exercise is simply to concentrate on what's happening while you make love. *Do not* allow yourself to have an orgasm. Instead, see what the contact of your partner's skin against your own feels like. Soak up the pleasure like a sponge. Actively keep your mind tuned to the present. See what happens when you merely relax and enjoy the sensations. Peggy had been separated for eight months from her husband, with whom she had been orgasmic. Although she had slept with a number of other men since the separation she had been unable to reach orgasm with any of them. She thought it might be guilt over leaving her husband or some other emotion that she wasn't aware of; she simply couldn't figure out the situation. When she entered the group she was involved with a lover whom she had known before she met her husband. She felt comfortable with him and had even been orgasmic with him some ten years earlier. Now she was at a total loss as to how to overcome the block. In the first session we instructed the women to attend to the sensations of the moment and forget about orgasm. For the first time in eight months Peggy had an orgasm with a partner, and continued to experience orgasm regularly thereafter. It appears that all she needed was permission to relax and enjoy sex for enjoyment's sake; then, free of anxiety and pressure, orgasm occurred.

Find a two-week stretch when you will be able to set aside an hour each day to do Partner Exercises 2–10. Masters and Johnson advocate a ban on intercourse during the time it takes to complete the initial few partner exploration assignments. I also encourage a ban on orgasms, even through masturbation.

During the days it takes to accomplish the first few partner exercises, try to forget that both intercourse and orgasm exist. Discuss the no orgasms/no intercourse ban with your partner. The ban should last for less than one week if you do the exercises daily. Deciding not to have intercourse or orgasms can help relieve the anxiety and concern that surround sex in which intercourse is the defined goal. Also, preventing orgasmic release while concurrently participating in erotic and sensual activities will help keep you in a sexual mood and maintain a high level of sexual arousal, even though it may prove to be a bit frustrating.

Although your partner cannot have intercourse with you, there is no reason why he cannot have orgasms. The procedure is not designed as punishment for a supportive lover. You can bring your partner to orgasm orally or manually, or your partner can stimulate himself to orgasm after an exercise is completed. The two of you can decide ahead of time how you want to work this out. Gloria and her husband decided that if he wanted her to manually stimulate him to orgasm after they had completed an assignment, she would do so. Whereas Betty and her husband agreed that they both could benefit from the exercises; he was willing to share the ground rules that she was going to abide by—no intercourse and no orgasm until later.

Couples sometimes break this no intercourse/no orgasms rule soon after they begin working on the assignments. Some women complained that their partners insisted on intercourse and they felt they had to acquiesce, or they themselves initiated coitus because they felt guilty. Since intercourse at this early stage rarely results in orgasm, the woman is frequently left feeling angry and resentful toward her partner for not caring about her needs. But remember, she agreed to participate. She could have refused and her partner could have achieved release in another manner.

Other women break the rule because they feel so aroused that they are sure they'll have an orgasm if they have intercourse *this* time. They usually don't and then are doubly disappointed. One or two experiences of feeling aroused is usually not sufficient to reverse past negative patterns. As soon as intercourse begins, the old worries and concerns generally come flooding back.

If you do break the rule and negative results occur, don't be concerned; just backtrack and begin over again, hopefully with greater resolve to follow the instructions more carefully.

Full body touching is usually very important to women, often more important in terms of sexual response than for most men. However, being attuned to the dimension of touch can greatly enhance a man's sexual experience, too. Women often complain that their partners do not spend enough time touching their bodies and genitals before intercourse begins. Lydia and Ellen both resented being awakened in the middle of the night for lovemaking because their partners would start directly with intercourse, with no preliminaries. Ellen claimed that having her mother rub salve on her chest when she had a cold was more sensual than having sex with her husband. Confining your activity to touching may seem like a regression when you're concerned about orgasm, but it really isn't. It is a way to get back to the initial building blocks of sexual excitement, a new way to approach sexual contact—a way to revisit adolescence, when just touching and kissing could send your body into a frenzy.

Partner Exercise 2 consists of spending two one-hour sessions revisiting the experience of touching by giving each other an information massage. All too many couples who have difficulties with their sexual relationship avoid touching one another—even nonsexual touch (touch whose primary goal is to produce pleasure but not necessarily arousal)—because of the expectation that touching has to lead to sex. This in itself creates physical distance between two people. Consequently, this exercise can provide an initial bridge in reestablishing feelings of closeness. Nonsexual touching can be a very enjoyable and sensuous experience and an important foundation to a relationship.

Begin with an area that is far from the center of your body: hands, feet, head, or face. Pick one area to be massaged, one that would be most pleasurable for you. For example, if you have very ticklish feet, a foot massage might not be a good choice. Your partner should pick one of these areas also, but it need not be the same choice as yours.

Decide who will give the first half-hour massage. You could do this by mutual decision or by flipping a coin. The point of the exercise is for the person who is doing the massaging to explore for the sake of whatever satisfaction he or she gets from it, *not to please the partner*. Don't worry about your technique—this is just for you. The exercise is designed so that the giver will relearn to appreciate the pleasure touching can have, in and of itself.

If your partner has chosen to receive a hand massage, pick up the hand gently and carefully. Caringly explore it in detail. Investigate nails, fingers, palm; lightly follow the vein structure and all the tiny lines on the skin. Using the fronts and backs of your hands to maintain physical contact, keep as much of your skin touching your partner's as possible. Explore the softer and rougher skin textures.

Apply some oil and massage more deeply, becoming familiar with the joints and the deeper muscles and bones. Remember, the person massaging is doing it for his or her own satisfaction, and to increase his or her own knowledge.

The person receiving the massage need only relax and enjoy it. This person has one responsibility, and that is to tell the person giving the massage to discontinue doing something if it is painful or distressing. You can make any pleasurable noises you might want to make, but during this exercise don't ask for anything unless it is to tell your partner that the massage is becoming uncomfortable. For those who are squeamish about being massaged, cut down the time spent, but do it for no longer than one half hour this first time.

After one person has finished giving the massage, switch places, making the receiver the giver. Angela's husband enjoyed giving his wife a massage, but he was uneasy about accepting one. He was very work-oriented and found considerable difficulty in allowing himself to relax and experience pleasure. In this case, they began with his receiving only a two-minute massage and built the time up slowly as he gradually learned to become a little more comfortable with receiving pleasure. In our culture, where the puritan work ethic is so strong, many of us feel guilty and lazy when we spend time giving and receiving pleasure. We are programmed always to have a purpose, to strive, to succeed, but not to relax and enjoy just being alive and feeling good.

Complete Partner Exercise 2 on at least two successive days (picking a different area to be massaged the second day) before moving on. After each session, sit down together for ten minutes and discuss what it was like to give and receive the massage. If you are finding the exercise particularly difficult to do, or if it is very uncomfortable for one or both of you, cut down the amount of time you spend in one session and extend the number of days, building up the time slowly until you can massage for one half hour with a fair degree of comfort. This is not a sexual exercise. It is designed to orient you toward touching for the pleasure of touching. *The Lover's Massage* videotape from the Alexander Institute[1] is a good reference if you desire to explore, in greater depth, massage as an activity.

Partner Exercise 3 is designed to go a little further. This activity will be aimed at awakening the whole body to sensations of touch. It will also provide an experience in which each of you has the opportunity to be alternately active and passive in a sexual situation. Furthermore, it will encourage open and direct communication about sensual stimulation.

This exercise is similar to the sensate focus advocated by Masters and Johnson.[2] Again, set aside an hour and decide who will go first. By this time you may have decided to take turns on succeeding days. Make sure the room is warm enough for you to be comfortable in the nude. Create a sensual atmosphere and setting. A sensual but not too filling meal may provide an enticing prelude.

The exercise is aimed at a total sensual body experience. Gather as many props as you can find—feathers, flannel, wool, velvet, satin, brushes, oils, powder. Explore your lover's body everywhere. Only breasts and genitals are off-limits. Often, the exploration of these two areas leads to the expectation of intercourse and may cause some women to feel tense or wary, thus preventing them from enjoying this activity fully.

The purpose of this exercise is not to arouse but to explore. Again, the person doing the exploring or the giving should do so for his or her own satisfaction primarily and for the partner's satisfaction only secondarily. The more the giver is enjoying the giving, the more pleasure the receiver is likely to glean.

The person on the receiving end need only relax and savor being touched. To enjoy sex more, there is value to learning to be temporarily selfish, to allow yourself to enjoy sensual pleasure with no other obligation. The additional requirement for this exercise, however, is for the receiver to let the giver know how things are going. The receiver can make some requests: "A little higher; harder; that tickles," etc. Noises indicating pleasure are valuable; nonverbal communication is very important. By placing your hand over your partner's you can help guide it to the specific area, pressure, or type of stroking you desire. Experiment with all these methods of communication.

The giver can also ask questions. Always be honest about what you want to do; never offer anything if you don't really want to do it.

Again, the receiver is responsible for letting the giver know whenever a certain touch is either irritating or not pleasurable. It is important that the giver not do anything he or she doesn't want to do. In real life, requests are often refused, so you need not feel obligated to consent just because a request has been made.

After a half hour, switch places. You get no extra points for giving longer than the assigned half hour, and your partner is not required to extend the massage session just because you did. Sticking to the time that you agreed on helps eliminate the resentment that one person may feel about giving more than his or her share and the indebtedness that the other person may then feel in return. Again, if one half hour apiece is too long, shorten the exercise time and build up slowly.

Maintaining the communication is essential, so after the exercise is over, discuss how each of you felt during the sensual body experience. What was it like to be assertive? Passive? What was it like to experience your partner as assertive or passive? Don't leave anything left unsaid, even if it only marginally relates to the experience. This is your time to communicate openly. Remember, still no intercourse and no orgasm for the woman.

Exercise 4 is called the sexological exercise and enables each of you to teach the other about your unique genital responses. Again, decide who will take the first turn. One of you will explore the other's genitals first visually and then by touching.

If your genitals are being explored, ask your partner to touch them in the same manner you did by yourself. Have your partner locate all the parts, then touch the various areas to see which are most sensitive. Have him hold the inner lips between his thumb and forefinger and gently tug to show the effect on the clitoris and clitoral hood that commonly occurs during intercourse. A finger could be inserted in the vagina, up to the end of the first joint of the index finger. Then the finger could be crooked slightly. If the vaginal opening is thought of in terms of a clock face, the part of the vagina closest to the abdomen, while the woman is lying on her back, would be twelve o'clock; firm, gentle pressure could be exerted on each "hour" of the clock. Are any of these points especially sensitive, pleasurable? If so, let your partner know. Contract the PC muscle when the finger is still inserted. Can your partner feel the pressure? Communicate how each part responds to touch and what kinds of touch feel best. A lubricant or oil should be used if the touching is experienced as irritating.

When it is your partner's turn to be explored, the illustrations in Masters and Johnson's *Human Sexual Response* could be used as a guide. First, examine his genitals visually, using sufficient light; the presence or absence of an erection makes no difference as far as carrying out the exercise, but an erection might change your partner's perception of the touching, since some areas of the penis might be more sensitive when erect. Which areas are most pleasurable when touched? The right side? The left? The midline underneath? The head? Which is preferred, a light movement of the fingers over the shaft or a more solid stroking that massages the structures below the skin? How hard can you squeeze the shaft near the glans without it hurting? Watch the muscles of the scrotum (the sac that holds the testicles) move when you stroke the inner thigh.

After you've explored each other's genitals, talk about what it was like to be explored and to explore. What did each of you like? Dislike? What did you learn from the experience?

At least four days of abstinence have probably now passed, and you may feel fairly aroused. The next exercise, the fifth, may be awkward, but it is important. It's time now to share everything you have learned about your own body by stimulating yourself in the presence of your partner.

Many people respond to this assignment with horror. "I couldn't do *that!*" "My partner would be disgusted." "I would be so embarrassed." However, Jack Rosenberg claims that "a couple that can learn to masturbate each other effectively with just the right timing for pleasure can accomplish a more creative and satisfying sexual union."[3] Since each of you has a unique way you like to be touched to reach orgasm, showing your partner how you stimulate yourself can teach him to be a better lover. Merely describing what you like may not be quite sufficient. Try to ignore any negative feelings and push beyond. At least broach the subject with your partner as a way to begin.

At first, when I realized that I would have to assign this exercise to the women in the groups, I told myself it wasn't necessary—we could skip this exercise in the progression. But I knew it was important for a woman be able to have an orgasm in the presence of her partner, and this could be an easy way to achieve it. So many women are afraid they'll look ugly or that their partners will be turned off, and these thoughts can inhibit expression of sexual feelings when a partner is present.

In the groups we discovered that doing this exercise is not necessarily difficult; in fact, some couples don't experience any shyness or discomfort at all. Others had to prepare themselves mentally for days before they could complete it.

I cannot emphasize enough how important it is to talk thoroughly about this assignment and your feelings about it before you begin. Talk about your discomfort. Just because you're not totally comfortable doesn't mean you have to discard the exercise. Together decide on the best way to carry out the assignment, so the two of you will be as much at ease as possible. You might prefer to masturbate side by side. Or, your partner can hold you while you masturbate or your partner can just watch if you find being touched a distraction. If it is really difficult, you might try having your partner turn away and not look at you the first time and then try again the next day with your partner watching.

Don't be surprised if you don't reach orgasm the first or second time you try this exercise. Many women need to masturbate in front of their partners a few times before they feel comfortable enough in the situation to let go.

The next exercise, Exercise 6, is designed to further open communication on sexual touching and to teach you to direct your partner in the type of touch that is most stimulating for you. Of course, there is no *one* kind of pressure or stroking that will be enjoyable at all times. The kind of touch that is stimulating will change with your level of excitement; this exercise helps you to practice keeping the communication lines open throughout the lovemaking experience.

Decide who will be massaged first. That person should lie on the bed on his or her back while the other person sits or lies beside. Once you are in position, have the person doing the touching run both of his or her hands over the body of the other person, while the partner being explored has his or her hands resting lightly over the explorer's hands. Betty found that she liked her partner to spread his fingers apart, and then when she placed her hands over his, she could fit her fingers between his and thus guide his hands and touch her own body at the same time. The explorer can explore everywhere, genitals included, but it's probably best to begin with other body areas first. Feel the skin textures, muscles, bones, and hair. Touch lightly with an almost feathery touch, then more firmly. Try circular stroking, figure eights, using the tips of your fingers and your whole hand. Explore your partner's erogenous areas: inner thighs, breasts and nipples, genitals, and the special areas uniquely sensitive to that individual such as ears, back of neck, stomach, feet, etc.

The person being explored should practice giving explicit reactions, both verbal and nonverbal, to the exploring partner. Let your partner know what feels good, where and how. Suggest some areas and types of touching you think you might enjoy. Don't settle for saying, "Everything you do feels good," but begin to state your preferences honestly. When your partner stimulates your genitals, use your own hands to guide your partner's both to the area you would like explored and the pressure and kind of stroking you prefer. When you switch roles to that of the exploring partner, try to use the information you learned from watching your lover's self-stimulation on the previous day. Can you duplicate that touch?

Your goal as receiver in Exercise 6 is to enjoy the stimulation and communicate your likes and dislikes to your partner. If you feel very aroused, somehow let your partner know that and explore further with the kinds of touching that might lead to orgasm. You may want to join your partner in exploring your own body by giving yourself the kind of stimulation that can result in climax.

A sexual relationship can be so much more rewarding if there are no rules and regulations restricting touching. Many couples subscribe to the rule: I touch only your genitals and you touch only mine. However, when both people can touch their partner and themselves as well, sexual enjoyment can be doubled. Nobody "gives" anybody else an orgasm—it's a mutual process.

The next exercise, Exercise 7, consists of transforming what has always been condescendingly labeled "foreplay" into a sexual experience that is important in itself. The ban on intercourse remains during this exercise. Tomorrow the exercise will include intercourse, but today it is essential to omit it.

Intercourse has always been considered "real sex" while "foreplay" has been a preliminary—something done primarily for the woman's pleasure. The touching, the manual and oral stimulation that precedes intercourse, is extremely pleasurable for most women, but men find it equally enjoyable once they cease to see it as a chore dutifully performed for a partner's benefit. Once men are relieved of some of the performance pressure that has historically been heaped upon them, they, too, can relax, be passive, and enjoy having their entire bodies stimulated.

Set aside an hour to elaborate on all the kinds of stimulation that precede and follow intercourse. While you and your partner are lying together, take turns being aggressive and passive; also stimulate each other simultaneously. Be as creative as you'd like to be. Possibly enact some of the fantasies you may have had or elaborate on all the kinds of caressing you enjoy. An hour is a fairly long time, so relax and move slowly. Enjoy the process—make the process the goal. Keep the communication lines open as to what feels good.

Again, orgasm is not the goal. If it happens, that's fine, but don't strive for it. Eventually orgasm will occur—usually after you have introduced changes in the lovemaking that make the experience a more exciting one for you so the stimulation can build.

Learning to appreciate and respond to sexual pleasure is analogous to learning to appreciate and respond to a piece of music. The first time you listen to a certain piano concerto, you may respond at one level. With future listening experiences, melodies, contrasts, and various nuances that were not noticed the first time become apparent. Then you can begin to respond to the piece at a different level. Of course, if while you're listening to the music you're also attending to the traffic noise outside, thinking about the grocery bill, or wondering how the piece will end, you won't be able to enjoy the experience as it is unfolding. The same holds true for sexual appreciation. Appreciating and responding to sexual stimulation requires devoting more time to sexual interaction, becoming more comfortable communicating to your partner about the kind of touch you like, and focusing on the touch and pleasure as opposed to the orgasm. Consequently, it may be necessary to practice each exercise a number of times with your partner before orgasm results.

The next exercise, Exercise 8, includes everything that has taken place before, plus intercourse. By this time each of you should have learned a great deal about the kind of stimulation that the other prefers. During this exercise, the communication lines should remain open as usual. Remember that you have a full hour to devote to the lovemaking, so there is no need to rush right into intercourse.

Only when you are highly aroused and feel you are ready to begin having intercourse should you let your partner know. Then, get into the female astride position. In this position, the man lies stretched out on his back between your legs as you kneel over him, vagina directly above his penis. Your face can be facing his head or feet. Then insert his penis. At this point, your level of sexual excitement may decline, but it is not a cause for concern. Once effective stimulation is begun again, the level of excitement will generally rise once again.

For this part of the exercise, it is important that your partner remain relatively inactive. It is up to you to control the speed and manner of thrusting by moving your pelvis up and down, back and forth, or in a circular motion, a movement some women find particularly stimulating. At the same time, consistently and continuously stimulate your clitoral area with your fingers or with a vibrator. Assume total control of the sex act. Don't expect to have an orgasm, just enjoy the pleasure of having your vaginal and clitoral areas stimulated at the same time.

Most women automatically make two assumptions. The first is that their actions are interfering with their partner's pleasure. The best way to check this out is to ask. Samantha was constantly asking her partner if he was enjoying pleasing her and was amazed to find that he was. Finally she realized that her assumption was an excuse because she felt that *she* didn't deserve all the attention and pleasure. It's good to keep in mind that your partner probably enjoys giving you pleasure as much as you enjoy giving your partner pleasure.

Your partner may be concerned that he will have an orgasm before you do and may try to hold back, but he need not. Rather, tell him to just relax and concentrate on the sensations he feels in his penis and if an orgasm approaches, let it take over. If this happens there is no reason for you to stop and consider the exercise over. In many cases the man is capable of maintaining a partial or even full erection if pelvic movement is sustained. But even if the erection is totally lost, you can continue to move slowly—not enough to cause his penis to come out, but enough to enjoy feeling it while continuing the clitoral stimulation. An orgasm can still be experienced with your partner inside, even if his penis is not erect. If he comes first, you may find yourself more able to relax and enjoy your own stimulation once the feeling of responsibility for your partner's pleasure is eliminated.

The second and more pervasive assumption women make is that it is taking too long to climax—a common concern if you experience difficulty reaching orgasm. And, ironically, as soon as you begin worrying about how long it is taking, it takes even longer. Louise used to blame her husband for the short duration of their lovemaking. But then she realized that it was her own fear the feelings wouldn't come that was causing her to hurry the experience. Beth would get aroused and then would feel she had had her quota of time and would turn her attention back to her husband. Both women used worrying about time as a way to terminate their own pleasure and cut off orgasm.

A woman's orgasm takes time, and when a woman is first learning, it may take even longer. Gebhard found that among couples who regularly spend twenty-one minutes or longer on foreplay, only 7.7 percent of the women failed to reach orgasm.[4] Relaxed and lengthy lovemaking can greatly enhance a woman's sexual experience. So before you begin making love, set aside sufficient time. Place a clock where you can see it easily; you'll be amazed at how slowly an hour of lovemaking passes.

Continue the stimulation in an uninterrupted manner for as long as is necessary for orgasm to occur. If you feel frustrated at some point, relax and just hold each other, or do whatever relaxes you until the frustration subsides. Remember, having an orgasm the first time through self-stimulation took time. Having it with a partner takes a while, too. It took Sarah one and a quarter hours the first time. The duration does get shorter with practice, as the feelings become more familiar.

If this exercise doesn't work the first time, don't be concerned. Repeat it over the next few days with whatever variations you prefer. You may have to practice this technique a number of times before you are successful. There is no rush. The only crucial part is that you continuously stimulate yourself while your partner's penis is inserted.

There are other positions that can be devised that afford access to the clitoral area during intercourse. These include: (1) the woman kneeling and the man, also kneeling, and entering her vagina from the rear; (2) the lateral position, in which the man lies on his side with the woman lying parallel to him, her back against his front and his bottom leg between her legs; (3) an X-shaped position in which the man lies on his side, and the woman sits perpendicular to him, with her legs flexed over his side, with the penis and vagina in proximity.

Once orgasm with your partner's penis inserted has occurred, you may still be interested in helping your lover learn to stimulate you manually to orgasm. You may want your partner to be more active, and he may want to be more involved as well.

The next exercise, Exercise 9, involves teaching your partner to stimulate your clitoral area manually. This requires a gradual approach for two reasons. First, your partner cannot know instantly what would be most pleasurable, as you know when you stimulate yourself, and so he may not be immediately aware of what you want at a particular moment. It is up to you to communicate this as the lovemaking proceeds. Second, it takes some time to get used to the type of stimulation your lover provides because it will be as individual to that person as your likes and dislikes are to you. Try to have your partner adjust his technique to become more compatible with your preferences, and also try to accommodate your responses to the stimulation afforded by your partner.

In this exercise, decide how much time you want your partner to spend stimulating you. It might be as short as two minutes the first time, or as long as an hour. Set aside a comfortable time period. The amount of time can be gradually increased with each succeeding practice session. Then guide your partner by putting your hands over his. Your lover will have seen how you stimulate yourself and will already have a basic idea of how to touch you, but you may have to supply the specifics. What feels good may change as your level of excitement increases.

Sarah asked her boyfriend Joe if he would devote three hours to stimulating her because that was how long she thought it would take for her to reach orgasm. She tried Kegeling while he stimulated her, and various fantasies. Finally she began concentrating on the pleasure she was feeling and then pretended that the feelings were those of orgasm. No sooner did she pretend orgasm was occurring than one actually did. Joe felt great about it and said, "It only took one and a quarter hours. We have lots of time left, let's do it again."

In the last exercise, Exercise 10, your partner applies the clitoral stimulation during intercourse. This exercise is last because it may be more difficult to be orgasmic when your partner is controlling the stimulation. It is not last because it is best; the only measure of what is best is the amount of satisfaction derived from a sexual experience. The positions described for Exercise 9 are applicable to this exercise. The only prerequisite for a particular position is that your clitoral area be available for manual stimulation. Begin intercourse only after you feel very aroused and close to orgasm. Your partner should continue to stimulate you in an uninterrupted manner and with an intensity that you find arousing.

I have consciously left out exercises which focus on orgasm without direct clitoral stimulation because for many women this is not possible. However, after you have progressed this far, you may choose to stop direct clitoral stimulation just short of orgasm to see if the penile thrusting is sufficient. If your arousal level begins dropping, you can simply reinstate the clitoral stimulation.

After Exercise 5, when orgasm is again permitted, it is important to continue the masturbation exercises between partner sessions. Being sexually responsive requires both technique and practice. As indicated in Chapter 9, the closer the masturbation positions and activities approximate those employed during lovemaking, the easier it will be to experience orgasm with a partner.

Remember, learning these procedures takes time. The majority of women in the groups required three to eight months of practicing the exercises—which they integrated into their usual lovemaking—before they were comfortably orgasmic with a lover.

The activities in this chapter have been directed toward restructuring your sexual relationship to meet needs expressed by many women. Most women find it enjoyable to have an orgasm at some time during lovemaking, but when or how the climax is achieved is not important. Even having an orgasm at all may sometimes be unimportant. You may feel tired or preoccupied and just being sexually close may provide sufficient comfort.

Some women need to spend considerable time in a relationship and get to know a partner fairly well before feeling free to express sexual preferences and sexual feelings. A number of women in the groups changed their attitudes toward their partners and lovemaking as a result of the group learning experience. Cindy lost interest in casual affairs and now feels strongly that the man she is interested in should be a considerate lover; she is interested in quality rather than quantity.

Changing your orgasmic responsivity with a partner takes not only time but also motivation. If either is lacking, and a haphazard approach to the process results, chances for success are lessened. Basic attitudes about sexuality change only over time and with the positive reinforcement of satisfying sexual experiences. The more successful sexual encounters you have, the more likely you are to expect a satisfying experience the next time and hence have it materialize. Caring, loving, being intimate and sexual all require sensitivity to the other person, and honest communication. It is both as easy and as difficult as that.

For more information on increasing desire and orgasm with a partner please read *For Each Other: Sharing Sexual Intimacy*, which I wrote as a sequel to this book.

13: Sexual Expansion

Expansion and innovation in your sexuality can result in a heightening of interest and pleasure, whether or not the various options always lead to orgasm. Depending upon the individual, expansion can occur in many directions: innovative coital techniques, innovative noncoital techniques, increased frequency of sex, integration of sexual paraphernalia, new sexual partners, partners of the same sex, etc. Sexual relationships can expand and grow in breadth and in depth. The important thing is to begin to express your sexuality more freely within the confines of the sexual boundaries in which you feel comfortable—to be able to explore further while still observing whatever moral, religious, intuitive, or common-sense feelings you have about sex.

An easy way to begin sexual expansion is to carry out a one-time experiment with something new and different for the sheer pleasure of trying it. The innovation need not be monumental. An interesting touch, no matter how small, can enhance sexual interaction. *Turn Ons: Pleasing Yourself While You Please Your Lover* contains fifty sexual innovations illustrated with erotic vignettes.

Nina experimented by initiating a shower with her husband; both soaped and washed each other in an erotic manner.

This was the first time she had ever initiated anything having to do with sex. She was pleased with the results and her husband was delighted. Sherry changed the furniture in the bedroom around to create a more sensual setting. Evelyn and her husband spent one night in a motel so they could feel really free from their children; she could then experiment with making as much noise during lovemaking as she wanted. Male and female stripteases, sensuous meals by candlelight, or even parking and necking can provide new sensual experiences.

Or, try changing roles. One night one partner could take complete charge; the other partner could do so the next time. Do you have any fears about being the initiator? If so, discuss them with your partner ahead of time. Simply bringing the fears into the open can make them less ominous.

Fantasies could be shared before or during lovemaking. Explicit sexual conversation can be very arousing for some people. Cindy told the group that she really enjoyed using four-letter words during sex.

Despite old laws remaining on the books that define oral sex as a perversion punishable by a prison term, a recent study found that around 80 percent of men and women with at least some college education and born after 1958 had practiced cunnilingus (the term for oral contact with the female genitals) and/or fellatio (the equivalent term for oral contact with the penis).[1] Obviously very few of the people interviewed are concerned about the legality of the practice; today it is very rare for anyone to be arrested and punished for participating in oral sex. Clearly, if so many people find oral sex enjoyable and sexually satisfying, and since there is no evidence that it is harmful, it should not be considered a crime. In many states it is in fact no longer considered illegal, but sexual mores change very slowly.

Many women find cunnilingus highly stimulating for a

number of reasons. First of all, as with manual stimulation, direct clitoral stimulation is provided, but this stimulation is much softer and gentler than that offered manually; also, saliva acts as a natural lubricant. In addition, oral sex leaves the hands free to stimulate other sexually responsive areas such as the breasts, thighs, and G-spot. The G-spot is an area on the front wall about a half finger's length into the vaginal opening. Some women enjoy the experience of having the tips of their partner's middle and forefingers pressing into this G-spot area in a rhythmic fashion during cunnilingus.

Nevertheless, many women dislike oral sex because they have negative feelings about their genitals. Women who consider their genitals "dirty" may expect their partner to feel the same way. Because of this expectation, these women cannot allow themselves to relax and enjoy the stimulation; instead, they protect their partner from this "distasteful" experience. But you don't have to protect your partner. You can ask him whether or not he finds oral contact with your genitals pleasant. Some men, as well as some women, may indeed be uncomfortable with oral sex and may need a period of time to adjust to this activity; others may not want to undertake it at all. But many find oral sex extremely pleasurable.

Jane had to overcome the feeling that oral sex was degrading to the person doing it. She always stopped her husband because she felt that performing oral sex put him in an unmanly position. Debbie, who was in a lesbian relationship, hesitated to participate in oral sex for fear that she would not be good at it. After seeing *Behind the Green Door*, a pornographic film, Debbie and her lover talked about oral sex. Between the movie and the discussion, Debbie became comfortable with the idea.

A woman may find it unpleasant for a partner to ejaculate in her mouth, while others enjoy the sensation. If this experience is uncomfortable for you, but you enjoy fellatio, work out a signal with your partner so that he can warn you just before he expects ejaculation to occur. Some couples find that a tap on the woman's head at the appropriate moment can solve this problem.

When you first begin to explore oral sex, it is advisable to do so slowly. Talk about it with your partner; share your feelings together before you begin. Take a bath or shower together as a prelude to the experience. In this way, you may feel more secure about the cleanliness of your genitals and those of your partner. Decide ahead of time that if either of you becomes ill at ease, that person will communicate the discomfort to the other and both of you will stop and return to more familiar lovemaking techniques.

Make sure that you assume a comfortable position. Begin by kissing the stomach and thighs. For the first time, it may be best to just brush your mouth across your partner's genitals. Then expand the time slowly. Kathy Kelly, in her unpublished "Radical Sex Manual," suggests, "Buildup is important. Slightly increase the pressure and the speed of stimulation . . ."[2] Then maintain a steady uninterrupted rhythm of stimulation once you begin experiencing an intensity and a pressure which you find arousing.

A variety of coital positions can also enhance one's sex life; however, it is important to find positions that are not uncomfortable for either partner. A position favored by one partner may not be the favorite of the other, but couples are free to employ several different intercourse positions during one session of lovemaking. Some positions may be better if the woman wants to touch her clitoris herself and others if her partner applies the stimulation. Rear entry positions often afford greater stimulation of the G-spot area.

The anal area can be highly erogenous; many women enjoy

oral as well as manual stimulation of the anus. Anal intercourse can be enjoyable although it is not very widely practiced among heterosexual couples. A recent study found that only 7 to 13 percent of couples in long-term relationships had had anal intercourse in the previous year.[3]

The anal sphincter muscle is quite strong and may not be penetrated easily at first. The "missionary" position, in which the woman is on her back with her knees or legs raised, making the anus accessible to the penis, may be a good position to begin with. A lubricant can facilitate the process. A lubricated condom both lubricates the anal entrance and protects the male's urethra against infection by any bacteria that may be present in the woman's rectum.

Once in this position the penis can be inserted slowly. Many women prefer the male to be passive at the beginning so that the woman can control both the rate of insertion and the thrusting movements. Later, the woman may be comfortable with her partner taking a more active role. Hygienically, it is essential that the male not insert his penis or fingers in the vagina without washing thoroughly after anal intercourse or anal play, because certain bacteria in the rectum when spread to the vagina can cause vaginal infections.

There are a number of sexual lifestyles that this book has not dealt with explicitly, but I hope have been implied: premarital sex, extramarital sex, group sex, homosexuality, bisexuality, and abstinence are all options. It is important that each person is able to express his or her own needs without it being seen as a threat to another's individuality. It entails acceptance of one's own lifestyle without trying to forcibly impose it on others. The ability to say yes or no to things because a person wants to or doesn't want to participate, and not because some leaders of the society say it is right or wrong, can lead to a peaceful coexistence in which people are able to learn from one another. Alix Shulman expresses these feelings very well: "There are actually laws on the books in most states that define as 'unnatural' and therefore criminal any (sexual) position other than that of the woman on the bottom and the man on the top; laws that make oral sex a crime, though for some women it is the only way of achieving orgasm with another person; laws that make homosexuality a crime, though for some people it is the only acceptable way of loving."[4] These laws should be repealed, not necessarily because you personally may want to participate in these activities, but so that people who do will have the freedom to do so with others who feel similarly inclined. Whether or not you want to experiment with any of the aforementioned possibilities is up to you. For some women, trying sexual innovations may be like walking a tightrope; you have to follow your instincts and sense of adventure without shaking the rope so hard that you fall off. Once aware of your own internalized limits, you may find that moving slowly in new areas can offer great pleasure.

14: Sex and Pregnancy,
Menopause, and Aging

The female reproductive system is far more complex than the male's. Major hormonal disequilibrium occurs during puberty, pregnancy, and menopause. During these periods a woman is still a sexual creature, but the changes occurring within her body, which in turn profoundly affect her state of mind, her sense of security, and her happiness, may also have a profound effect upon her sexuality.

Sexuality during pregnancy has been only sparsely researched and most research divides the nine-month gestation period into three trimesters. Masters and Johnson's[1] research on 101 pregnant women, and the research by Solberg, Butler, and Wagner[2] on 250 women indicate a general loss of sexual desire by women during the first trimester. Of course, there are exceptions; some women are more erotically inclined. But in general, possibly because of the fatigue and nausea that sometimes accompany the early months of pregnancy, many women tend to lose interest in sex. Women also frequently complain of severe breast tenderness during sexual excitation at this point.[3] A fear of injury to the fetus during intercourse is another reason cited by many women for cutting back on sexual activity.

It is true that women with a history of miscarriage during

the first trimester should refrain from sexual activities, including masturbation, but if this history is not present and there is no abdominal pain or bleeding, there is generally no physical reason not to enjoy sex. However, since pregnancy often causes a real drain on the woman's body, some women may not have the energy to be sexually active, especially if they have other children to care for or a job commitment to fulfill.

Some women experience an increase in sexual desire during the second trimester,[4] but a number of studies show a progressive decline in the frequency of intercourse as the pregnancy progresses.[5] However, exceptions to the general trend were apparent, indicating again the highly individualistic relationship between pregnancy and sex.[6] For example, Tina, who during her fourth and fifth months had no interest in partner sex and who experienced considerable discomfort with intercourse, found that her desire and frequency of masturbation increased markedly.

Masters and Johnson noted some physiological differences in the sexual response cycle between pregnant and nonpregnant women. First, lubrication generally develops more rapidly and in greater quantity when a woman is pregnant.[7] Orgasms tend to be as satisfying or more so during the second stage of pregnancy, and it is not uncommon for women to become orgasmic, or multiply orgasmic, for the first time, during and/or after pregnancy.[8] This change may be the result of the increased vascularity in the pelvic area that develops to nourish the fetus.[9]

Because of the increased vascularity, and increased blood supply, the pelvis area can become very congested during sexual excitement—as a consequence, even though the woman experiences a satisfying orgasm, that orgasm may fail to resolve sexual tension completely. Therefore, the resolution phase may take a considerable period of time.[10]

During the last trimester of pregnancy, Solbert et al. again find decreased sexual activity and decreased frequency of orgasm resulting from coitus.[11] This effect may be due to the discomfort of an advanced pregnancy or the awkwardness of coitus in addition to the fear of injuring the fetus or causing a premature birth.[12] Or it could simply be the result of a belief that sex should be discontinued during this period.

Sexual activity during the last six weeks or month of pregnancy appears to be the major point of controversy. Masters and Johnson[13] and the Sex Information and Education Council of the United States (SIECUS)[14] agree that decisions about sexual abstinence should be made in an individualized manner, with the advice of a physician. There is no real evidence that orgasms occurring during the last trimester cause premature births.[15] The consensus is that there is no reason for abstinence from sexual activities during the last months of pregnancy for any reason other than the woman's own physical discomfort, providing that she is free of pelvic or abdominal pain, uterine bleeding, ruptured membranes which can cause infection to mother and child, actual labor, and individual problems accompanying the last weeks of pregnancy.[16] In the case of individual problems, a physician may require abstinence from all sexual activity which leads to orgasm—including masturbation. If intercourse is thought to be unwise, check with your physician to see whether other sexual activities are permissible.

Some women use doctors' orders to legitimize their lack of desire, a lack which is totally normal and frequently felt by pregnant women, and a lack which really requires no justification. The extensive physical and hormonal changes occurring during pregnancy are highly individual, and each woman responds according to her overall physical and psychological makeup. There is no "normal" response. Some women desire sex more often than before pregnancy and some less often. Some find it more satisfying and some less so. Solbert et al. indicate, however, that a lack of desire is more likely to occur in women who do not normally experience orgasm with partner sexual activity.[17]

The woman's behavior is not the only cause for reduced sexual activity. The male partner may lose sexual interest during his partner's pregnancy. Common reasons include concern for the expectant mother's physical comfort, fear of injuring the fetus, and sometimes aversion to the physical appearance of the pregnant woman.[18] It is important for men to be aware of the tremendous physiological drain of pregnancy, and also of the mental preparations for child rearing which may be diminishing the woman's sexual interest. In general, however, her need for intimacy and caring, if not sex, is often greater during this period than at other times.

During the advanced stages of pregnancy, it is helpful to keep in mind many of the previously mentioned noncoital techniques and positions which can be used for more pleasurable, and less awkward and uncomfortable, sexual activity. The woman astride position, the X-shaped position, and all the rear-entry positions can help to alleviate discomfort. Manual stimulation and oral sex can provide excellent means for achieving sexual pleasure if orgasm is not prohibited by your physician. With oral sex, make sure that no air is blown into the vagina, because air bubbles entering the uterus during pregnancy can cause an embolism which may prove fatal to the fetus and the mother.[19]

The important thing to realize is that you can continue to be sexual if you want to be so long as your physician finds no concrete reasons to prohibit sexual activity. Having a couple refrain from sexual activity during a period in which both are going through considerable changes and may really desire and require the intimacy that sex provides may put an unnecessary strain on the partners and on the relationship.

Authorities also disagree about the need for a lengthy period of sexual abstinence after birth. It depends upon the individual woman's situation, her level of sexual desire, and especially her rate of healing and recovery from the delivery.[20] Bleeding should have ceased, although a brownish discharge may persist and can often be disregarded.[21] Unfortunately, the sexual structures may have been damaged by careless obstetrical handling and many women unnecessarily experience lasting pain with intercourse as the result. Practicing the Kegel exercises can promote healing and tightening of the vagina after delivery and nursing often assists the recovery process. Women generally tend to experience more intense and satisfying orgasms after their first pregnancy and this change appears to be permanent.[22]

The research of Masters and Johnson indicates that nursing mothers show a more rapid return to being sexually interested than non-nursing mothers.[23] The relatively rapid revival of sexual interest suggests that nursing may promote a faster recovery because of the accompanying uterine contractions; these contractions may help stop the bleeding and return the uterus to its normal state more quickly.[24] Some sensual-sexual feelings can accompany the act of nursing. Some women have even experienced orgasm while nursing their infants.[25] In the past many women have felt guilty or abnormal because of these perfectly normal sensual feelings.[26]

One problem is that women are made to feel embarrassed about nursing, embarrassed to expose a breast in public, embarrassed if the nursing feels pleasurable, and especially embarrassed if nursing is continued past early infancy.

Despite prevailing folk wisdom, it should be noted that nursing is not a dependable contraceptive even though it can, in many cases, retard ovulation for a considerable period of time. Some birth control method should be instituted immediately after the baby's birth if pregnancy is not desired right away.

Sexual activity in the advancing years is another common source of concern for women. Menopause can be a time of considerable mental conflict as well as physical discomfort for many women. Not only do changes in the woman's hormone balance make it obvious that her reproductive years are over, but these changes may make her feel as if her youth has ended and with it her femininity, attractiveness, and desirability as a sexual partner. However, being older and experienced and without the responsibility of children can give a woman a new-found freedom to continue to explore and grow sexually. Aging need not bring a decline in spirit, but a spirit tempered by experience. The pace may be slower, but the enjoyment need not be less.

Our culture's emphasis on youth and beauty causes older women an unnecessary insecurity. Darlene was nearing fifty and still found her husband very sexy, his slight paunch notwithstanding. He found her equally desirable, but she feared that her sexual drive would lessen after menopause; although she enjoyed being affectionate, she was so afraid that she would lose her sexual interest that she avoided the whole issue by getting out of bed first in the morning or avoiding sex in other ways in order not to confront what she thought was inevitable. In the group, we simply corrected this misapprehension. Now she is initiating sex more often and is delighted to find that she enjoys it as much as before. It was only her fear of not being sexual as she grew older that diminished her enjoyment—not the physiological fact of aging.

As women age, lubrication may be diminished or slower in developing and the intensity and duration of orgasm may be reduced. But other problems can be helped by hormone therapy and by continued, regular sexual activity.

Unfortunately, the normal slowing down of sexual responses in both the older man and woman may affect a man's feeling of masculinity. As a result, his desire for sex may decrease as he sees his erection forming more slowly and with less firmness. However, sexual activity need not cease or even radically diminish as a man ages. If he is slow to reach erection, he can stimulate his partner manually and orally and the couple can continue to indulge in mutually satisfying lovemaking. As a matter of fact, pleasure may increase for both, since more time is needed for caressing and stimulating each other in order to attain high levels of excitement.

The experience of orgasm is not essential to the enjoyment of sex play. Many older couples are capable of enjoying sex that does not result in orgasm each time. It only seems fair that the slow, relaxed pleasure of sex should be one of the benefits of growing older.

Women undergoing menopausal changes often find the fatigue, irritability, headaches, hot flashes, and nervousness enough of a drain to make them lose interest in sex. However, hormone therapy can reduce these discomforts and help to reestablish sexual interest. It can also help if intercourse is painful. Vaginal pain sometimes results from lack of estrogen. This deficiency causes the vaginal walls to become thin, providing less protection for the bladder and urethra during intercourse and thus causing a burning sensation and frequently the need to urinate following intercourse. Also, a lack of hormones reduces the expansibility of the vagina, which may make accommodating the penis uncomfortable. A lubricant can be helpful in supplying sufficient lubrication. In *The Pause: Positive Approaches to Menopause*, I have outlined numerous hormonal and alternative approaches to relieving sexual and other symptoms that may accompany menopause.

However, the best preventative for sexual discomfort as we age is an active sex life, both masturbation and/or intercourse. Masters and Johnson found that women who engaged in intercourse on the average of once or twice a week had little difficulty producing sufficient lubrication and experienced little or no discomfort with sex as compared to women with a less active sex life.[27] However, it is also important to recognize the reaction of many older women who never or only rarely enjoyed sex and who may be thoroughly relieved finally to be able to use menopause or a hysterectomy as a reason to avoid sex altogether.

One perplexing problem that faces many older women who desire sexual activity is a lack of available sexual partners. Because women live longer than men, they are more likely to find themselves without sexual partners in later years. One eighty-seven-year-old great-grandmother asked me what she could do about her considerable sex drive, since she had no current sexual partner. For her and other older women in similar situations, self-stimulation can be very important in providing a regular and satisfying release of sexual tensions.

15: Your Responsibility to Your Body

While this book specifically addresses sexuality, it is in essence speaking to the larger subject of how women can take responsibility for themselves. Being responsible for oneself includes taking care of one's body and general health.

The information in this chapter is not new. The media are constantly bombarding us with messages urging preventative health measures, but we frequently don't heed these messages—sometimes because we don't consider ourselves important enough to take adequate health precautions.

For example, taking care not to get pregnant if you don't want a child is essential. Birth control is now readily and inexpensively available in this country through county public health services and Planned Parenthood—yet many women are seeking abortions for unplanned pregnancies.

Abortions are safer and more easily obtained today than ever before, but they can cause considerable mental anguish. All birth control methods seem to have their drawbacks, but generally speaking, they are probably more acceptable than an unwanted pregnancy or sexual abstinence. *Our Bodies, Ourselves* by the Boston Women's Health Book Collective gives an excellent description and sensitive presentation of the various birth control methods, providing information on how they work, their complications or drawbacks, and where they can be obtained.[1] You might refer to that book if you are considering birth control for the first time or if you are dissatisfied with your present contraceptive method.

Being aware of sexually transmitted diseases is especially important for any sexually active female. Contrary to myth, "nice girls" do get STDs. Sexually transmitted diseases attack males and females of all ages and all social classes. Sexual contact with a partner who harbors the disease is all that is needed for exposure. If you suspect that you have been exposed, see your doctor or visit a clinic.

The most common STDs are chlamydia, gonorrhea, herpes, syphilis, human papillomavirus (HPV) or genital warts, trichomoniasis, and human immunodeficiency virus (HIV), which causes acquired immunodeficiency syndrome (AIDS). The number of STDs has increased dramatically since the mid-1970s when I wrote the first version of this book. Then we mostly had to worry about gonorrhea, syphilis, and trichomoniasis. These last three venereal diseases might cause infertility, but all were curable if treated early enough. Now we have sexually transmitted diseases that can cause not only infertility, but also death. Some continue doing damage even after their symptoms have disappeared.

Chlamydia, a bacterial STD, is the most common STD around today. Unfortunately, approximately 75 percent of women will have no symptoms, and as a result of not being diagnosed, chlamydia can destroy the fallopian tubes, resulting in infertility.[2] Chlamydia is transmitted through direct contact of the infected mucous membranes of the genitals, mouth, or throat. A polymerase chain reaction (PCR) test can be used to diagnose the disease and the appropriate antibiotic can cure it.

Like chlamydia, gonorrhea is often silent and can cause infertility. Symptoms, when present, include burning with urination, and as gonorrhea becomes more advanced, it can cause pelvic pain, fever, and nausea. Like chlamydia, it is transmitted through direct contact with the infected mucous membranes of the genitals, mouth, or throat. A culture test can diagnose the disease and penicillin or a combination of antibiotics will eradicate it.

Herpes is a very widespread viral STD. A herpes outbreak generally consists of one or more sores on the genitals, buttocks, thighs, or anal area, which can sting, burn, or itch. You may also experience a fever and flu-like symptoms as well as a vaginal discharge or swollen glands in the groin. The virus is transmitted through direct contact with a herpes sore or, in some cases, the genital secretions of a person whose virus is active but has produced no sores. A viral culture can be used to diagnose herpes. Acyclovir in pill or cream form can reduce symptoms, but most people with herpes continue to get outbreaks throughout their lives, especially during times of stress or illness.

Syphilis is one of the oldest bacterial venereal diseases. It often begins as a painless sore on or around the genitals and then may develop into a rash. Direct contact with a sore is necessary to contract the disease. A blood test will confirm diagnosis, and antibiotics are used to treat it. It is curable if treated in the early stages.

There are about twenty kinds of sexually transmitted genital warts (HPV). Since men often experience no symptoms with HPV, they can pass it around unwittingly. The disease is transmitted by direct genital skin-to-skin contact with an infected person, even if the warts are not visible. While most genital warts are benign, a couple types are thought to be related to cancer of the cervix. Nothing can completely get rid of the virus, but the warts themselves can be burned off with liquid nitrogen, electric current, or laser surgery.

Trichomoniasis is caused by a parasite that is transmitted through intercourse. It causes a heavy gray, greenish, or yellowish vaginal discharge. Looking at the discharge under a microscope can diagnose the disease and metronidazole is the drug that can cure trichomoniasis. But unless both partners are treated, the parasite will continue to be passed back and forth.

The human immunodeficiency virus (HIV) causes AIDS. HIV is spread through an exchange of infected blood or sexual fluids. A blood test can diagnose the disease, but there is no cure for HIV or AIDS, and AIDS can result in death.

Finally, women are far more susceptible than men to contracting sexually transmitted diseases and the diseases do more harm to our reproductive organs. Take care of yourself. To prevent all STDs, use latex condoms with the spermicide nonoxynol-9 *every time* you have sex until you are certain your partner is disease-free. If you use a lubricant with a condom, make sure it is water-based. A petroleum-based lubricant can weaken the latex.

Anyone who has an STD is responsible for notifying everyone with whom he or she has had recent sexual contact so that they can obtain testing and, if infected, treatment. Reporting contacts is a major step toward controlling the spread of STDs; there are no vaccines to protect us. Such vaccines are needed, but little has been done to develop them, in part because our culture has assumed that a sexually transmitted disease is appropriate punishment for those who insist upon what society considers "immoral sexual contact" (more than one sexual partner).

Until more money is spent on education, research, and preventative treatment, it is more important than ever for everyone who is not in a mutually monogamous relationship to protect himself or herself by using condoms with nonoxynol-9 100 percent of the time. Condoms provide the best protection available from contracting a sexually transmitted disease. For further information about STDs, your local public health service, community pharmacist, family planning agency, physician, school nurse, or free STD clinic should be contacted.

Vaginal infections are a very common source of discomfort for many women. The most common vaginal infections are yeast infections and trichomoniasis. Vaginal infections sometimes cause itching or burning. Yeast infections often result from unusual emotional stress, contraceptive pills, antibiotics, or excessive douching, all of which can alter the natural pH of the vagina, thereby providing the already present bacteria with a more conducive environment in which to thrive. Inserting yogurt into the vagina or a mildly acidic douche (two tablespoons of white vinegar to one quart warm water) can alleviate the problem, but if it persists, simple over-the-counter medication is generally effective.

If yeast infections recur, it might be beneficial to substitute cotton underpants for nylon and not wear clothes that are tightly fitted in the crotch area. Always urinate after intercourse, and, if all else fails, you may need to change your method of contraception, your diet, or certain factors in your emotional environment.

Vaginal infections are not generally as serious as sexually transmitted diseases, but they can be more uncomfortable. They should be attended to promptly.

Taking care of your sexual organs includes a Pap smear, a painless procedure to check for uterine cancer. This test should be done at least once a year, or more frequently if any irregular cells are found as a result of the test. Uterine cancer is not uncommon, but if diagnosed early, procedures less severe than a hysterectomy (the removal of the uterus) are possible, and the chance that the cancer will spread to other organs is greatly reduced. Through a regular and painless exam an untimely death can be prevented.

In addition to seeing your doctor for a once-a-year checkup, you must be responsible for examining your breasts every month. Don't wait for your physician to check your breasts only once a year. Lie on your back, lift your right arm over your head and examine your right breast thoroughly with your left hand. Massage the whole area deeply with circular motions. Reverse the position to examine your left breast. When you first begin to check your breasts, the natural and normal masses may scare you, but self-examination of the breasts following each period, when they are less grainy and lumpy, will familiarize you with the normal masses; then if an abnormal lump appears, you can have it immediately checked by a doctor. Only a small percentage of unusual breast lumps are cancerous. If you let a lump go too long and it is malignant, the cancerous cells can infect the lymphatic system and spread to other organs of your body. Early treatment is essential. Ignoring a lump will not make it go away. As difficult and scary as it is to face the possibility of having breast or uterine cancer, especially if it runs in your family, it is still essential to take these precautions.

Both women and men have a tendency to ignore or neglect medical problems that can become more severe the longer they are left untended. Some of us ignore our medical problems because we fear they might be serious. Others of us do so because we have received disagreeable or humiliating treatment by physicians in the past that has made us dread a physical and especially a pelvic exam. Unfortunately, many doctors are insensitive to the discomfort a woman feels, with her feet in stirrups and her crotch in full view. It seems, though, that the more exams we get the more we realize how routine it is for the doctor and the less embarrassing it is for us. However, if your physician uses cold speculums for pelvic examinations, despite your requests to warm them, or treats you harshly or disrespectfully, by all means change doctors. Don't let discomfort with a physician cause you to procrastinate about getting regular checkups.

Finding a competent doctor you like is extremely important, but often not easy. Gynecologists frequently disagree among themselves about appropriate treatment. I could cite hundreds of medical horror stories from ignored breast lumps to unnecessary hysterectomies in young women. Find a physician you trust—male or female, neither is infallible—and receive regular medical exams. Check on potential problems immediately. Make certain you understand what is happening. Demand information. Don't accept a hasty dismissal. If you are uncomfortable with the exam, or the doctor's diagnosis, or the treatment suggested, you have every right to another medical opinion. Millions of women deny the existence of physical ailments which only become worse over time. No one wants to be considered a complainer or a hysteric who gets excited about the least little thing. You may feel embarrassed if you consult a doctor and turn out to be *well* instead of dying. Also, it's natural to want to believe that there is nothing wrong, so we disregard our fears. However, it is important to complain when it comes to our physical health, for if we don't, no one else will.

Our lives are essentially our responsibility.

16: Bringing Up Children Sexually

Many women in the groups were concerned about what they could do so that their children, particularly their daughters, would not grow up with the same inhibitions and misconceptions about sex that had taken so much time and energy to reverse in themselves. Few good books have been written about the sexual education of children. Material is available carefully detailing how to explain reproductive matters and at what age information is appropriate, but very little has been researched or written about how to deal with children's natural curiosity about sexual matters. A few good books do exist: *It's Perfectly Normal*, by Robie Harris and illustrated by Michael Emberley; *The Period Book,* by Karen Gravelle; *Growing Up: It's a Girl Thing*, by Mavis Jukes and illustrated by Debbie Tilley; and *The What's Happening to My Body? Book for Boys*, by Lynda Madaras, Dane Saavedra, and Ralph Lopez.

Self-exploration is a natural part of the developmental process, and this includes a child's exploration of bodies—the mother's body, the father's body, friends' bodies, and the child's own body.

Would you like to have been brought up so that you were less inhibited and more sensual and sexual? How can we change things so our children can have a better experience? Child rearing is an individual matter and something with which each mother and father has to struggle. Perhaps this discussion will present a few options for you to explore further in your family.

All too frequently, children have been treated as innocent, asexual beings. But children most certainly are not asexual. All the sexual organs capable of providing pleasure are present, and children are sexual creatures, from birth. Theirs is not the same sexuality we know as adults, but it is nonetheless sexuality. The baby playing with your breast is at least sensual. The two-year-old who seductively crawls into bed between Mommy and Daddy is sexual, although not with the same explicit sexual intent of an adult. The five-year-old girl who dresses up and sits on her father's lap kissing him and asking him if he will marry her when she grows up is sexual. The seven-year-old who is masturbating, possibly even to orgasm, is sexual. The eight-year-old prancing around without any clothes on is sexual. These are children passing through learning stages on the way to becoming adult sexual beings. Some of their behavior represents a mimicking of Mommy or Daddy and some results from natural bodily curiosity, but it is all sexual.

A major problem in dealing with sexuality in children has been our own embarrassment and discomfort with sex. There has been a tendency to ignore children's sexual questions and gestures, a tendency to believe that we don't have to answer sexual questions because the child couldn't possibly know what she is asking. This denies the child's sexuality because of our own uneasiness. The result, of course, is that the child gets the message that she is asking improper questions, ones her mother doesn't like to hear, so the child's tendency is not to risk her mother's anger, keep quiet, and wonder silently to herself.

Meanwhile, the child feels embarrassment, shame, and remains ignorant about sex, and many reach adulthood and experience excessive sexual inhibitions, the absence of orgasm, or the experience of an unwanted pregnancy.

Open, honest, direct dealing with sexual questions or sexual curiosity in children is best. The child should be given information, with the parent frequently asking questions to determine if the child understands, if she has any further questions, if the information has disturbed or upset her, so the parent can correct any misconceptions from the beginning.

The biggest obstacle is dealing with issues that are not quite resolved in our own mind, while still trying to be honest. One mother accepted masturbation intellectually, but found the old fears and feelings of disgust or shame were evoked when her son played with his penis. She did not want to alarm him by forbidding him to touch himself, but she knew he would detect her discomfort if she told him that what he was doing was fine, while she was feeling otherwise. Children pick up mixed messages quickly and respond with confusion. They realize something is wrong, although they may not be sure exactly what. A parent's attempt to inform the child of more than one prevailing intellectual opinion while also directly expressing personal discomfort may be one way of dealing with unsettled issues. In that way at least the child knows exactly why a parent is uncomfortable. This particular woman said, "I know it feels good to play with your penis and it's OK, but it makes me uncomfortable when you do it here in the living room. I would feel much better if you would go into your bedroom where you can have privacy."

It is important for children to know that touching their sexual organs is supposed to feel good—that other people touch themselves and have similar sensations and the response is not abnormal or shameful; that sometimes a special feeling called orgasm can occur. It might be a good idea to say that the feelings are good feelings and should be enjoyed but possibly only in the privacy of one's own room, and when others aren't around. There are special rooms for many activities (kitchen, bathroom, etc.). Children are able to understand this.

Physical contact is essential for children. Studies show that children in orphanages who received adequate nourishment but were not held, cuddled, kissed, and caressed would often become ill.[1] But in our culture it is customary to discontinue physical contact as the child grows older, especially with sons. Then after marriage, miraculously, the two people who have been denied physical contact for years are supposed to be able to respond physically and emotionally without inhibitions—which was natural for them as children, but was trained out of them as they grew older.

Many of us grew up in families where touching was prohibited and so we tend to maintain a distance from our children. Others of us may find ourselves sexually aroused by our children, and these impulses may frighten us so much that we maintain physical distance in an effort to avoid the unacceptable sexual feelings and possibly even to protect our children from being the object of our sexual fantasies.

Sexual feelings or fantasies about one's children are normal. Many mothers in the groups reported having some such feelings at least occasionally. Children are sexual, warm, cuddly human beings—we can feel turned on and have the fantasies, but we don't have to act them out. Acting them out can be seriously detrimental to the child, while just having the fantasy is perfectly harmless.

Accurate information is important to curious youngsters. If your relationship is a close and caring one, and your child trusts you and feels comfortable with you, she will look to you for guidance and answers—especially in the early years. During adolescence things may change because of the adolescent's intense need for privacy and rebellion in order to establish herself as her own person. But if your relationship has been open until then, your daughter should have received the necessary information about sexuality before this difficult and conflicted time.

Information need not exceed the limits of the child's question. A child asks a question, but we may not be aware of exactly what it is she wishes to have explained. Seeing the world through a child's eyes, and knowing exactly what she wants to know, can be very hard for an adult. A good way to find out precisely what is confusing your daughter, which in turn will make it far easier to answer her question, is to ask what *she* thinks about it or how *she* thinks it works. This can radically simplify a seemingly all-encompassing question. For example, one three-and-a-half-year-old asked Diane, "How does a car work?" Diane's mind immediately raced to all the complexities of a combustion engine, most of which she really didn't understand herself. But before she jumped in over both their heads, Diane asked, "How do *you* think it works?" "Well, I *don't* think you push it with your feet," the child answered. This greatly simplified Diane's problem as she explained the absolute rudiments of a motor attached to the wheels that causes the car to move. If the child wants more information, she will usually ask further questions. Generally, children hear only as much as they are prepared to hear at a particular point in time and walk away when they become anxious or burdened with information they cannot handle. Always asking if the child understands or has further questions or is upset by something you have said can help weed out the child's misconceptions and keep disturbing information from festering within.

Using diagrams and pictures can sometimes clarify matters,

or just using words that a child will not misinterpret. A friend of mine was told at the age of five that babies came from an egg in Mommy's tummy that Daddy fertilized. For years she carried around the mental image of Daddy shoveling manure on a chicken egg sitting on top of Mommy's tummy.

Information about sex is generally met by children with embarrassment and giggles—especially at the beginning. Their reaction may make it even more difficult for us to sensitively answer their questions if we feel they are not serious or are ridiculing us, particularly when we are already experiencing discomfort trying to deal with the issue. Since children may pick up our discomfort or may already be aware that this is a private subject, and they may feel awkward and uneasy discussing sex even though they are starved for accurate information. However, as you begin to address their questions, children will generally quiet down and listen attentively.

There is no reason to keep children from knowing that sex is an enjoyable, pleasurable activity; that sex is for fun first and for babies second. It makes no sense to hide the physical side of a loving relationship. It is important for children to see their parents embrace, kiss, cuddle, and in general act affectionately toward one another. However, in our culture, this does not mean making love with the children as spectators or participants, though two- to four-year-olds have a fantastic ability to open unlocked doors at precisely the wrong moment. It might be a good idea to let your child know that you and Daddy make love in the privacy of your bedroom; that during that time you don't like to be disturbed and most questions and problems can wait until afterward. To treat sex with dignity and love rather than to shroud it in awkward and unspeakable mystery is an excellent way of instilling a child with a healthy attitude toward sex.

The pleasure sex provides can be acknowledged rather than ignored. Young girls and boys can be told about a girl's clitoris just as they are told about a boy's penis, so that when they accidentally discover this tiny but pleasurable organ, they don't feel like freaks. Alix Shulman wrote a lovely dialogue about explaining the difference between boys and girls:

> BOY: What's the difference between boys and girls?
>
> MOTHER: Mainly their sex organs. A boy has a penis and a girl has a clitoris.
>
> BOY: What's a clitoris?
>
> MOTHER: It's a tiny sensitive organ on a girl's body about where a penis is on a boy's body. It feels good to touch, like your penis. . . .
>
> BOY: What's it for?
>
> MOTHER: For making love, for pleasure. When people love each other, one of the ways they show it is by caressing one another's bodies, including their sex organs.
>
> BOY: How do girls pee?
>
> MOTHER: There's an opening below the clitoris for peeing. A man uses his penis for peeing, for making love, and for starting babies. Women have three separate places for these. . . . (and so on . . .)[2]

Children are innocent and curious. They know no guilt until others instill it in them, and sometimes it happens without parents even noticing. Sarah walked in on her four-and-a-half-year-old daughter while she was masturbating, and the child began to cry hysterically. She hated herself because she did this and made her mother promise not to tell anyone. Sarah had no idea how her daughter got these negative feelings at such a young age. She could not remember ever telling her daughter that it was bad to touch herself.

This illustration makes it only too clear how little control we actually have over what a child hears and sees outside the home. Unless given permission and positive messages about sex from their parents, children all too quickly receive negative sexual messages from society, religion, schools, friends, and relatives. Positive and accepting statements about sex, as opposed to the old oppressive messages, might make a difference later on. Landis et al. found that catching a child in the act of masturbation or making threatening statements about the act induces guilt, but has no effect on the frequency of masturbation. The child will continue to masturbate, but will also feel guilty about it.[3] Also, Kinsey's research indicates that a better sexual-orgasmic adjustment to marriage is more probable if the girl has experienced orgasm, by whatever means, prior to marriage.[4] These are good reasons not to discourage a daughter's masturbation.

Children's sexual exploration is like all other areas of exploration. For the child it is a way of learning about her environment and how to make a place for herself within it. Exploration includes urinating while standing up like a boy, wearing makeup like Mother, playing doctor with other boys and girls down the street, and exploring sexual feelings with a girlfriend. Physical and loving relationships between two or more girls or two or more boys is a very common and natural part of the growing-up process. It does not mean that the child is heterosexual, homosexual, or bisexual. Each child will become clear about his or her sexual orientation later on in life. As parents, our job is to enable our children to feel normal and unashamed about the expression of budding sexual feelings.

Perhaps the most important source of feelings toward sexuality and about a girl's own body comes from messages from her mother. If we approach life positively and freely, sharing our enthusiasm and love, and if we look beyond the traditional roles so confining for our daughters, then it is likely that our daughters will develop in less inhibited and more optimistic, self-sufficient, and independent ways.

17: Personal Liberation

What if you have assumed responsibility for your sexuality and followed the exercises in this book diligently, and still experience no progress in attaining sexual satisfaction? Hopefully, you are enjoying sex more now, even if you aren't orgasmic yet. However, what can you do now? One alternative is to begin the program a second time, especially if your first attempt was unsystematic. Beth's experience illustrates what you can do on your own. A month after the group ended, Beth wrote: "Though my sexual responses are far from secure, I did climax recently while being pleasured by Lee! This is a big first, the goal I had just about given up achieving. This, though I don't understand how it happened, tells me I'm on the right track. I will continue the exercises and homework as faithfully as possible, on the assumption that it was these things that led me to my initial success."

Still, even with time, the tools contained in this book may be insufficient to help you realize your sexual potential. But don't despair. If you have a clitoris, you can have an orgasm (except in extremely rare circumstances), but you may require individualized assistance. Or, you may want to get a physical exam if you suspect your testosterone level is too low or you are experiencing some other medical difficulty.

Sometimes a friend who is compassionate, or a small group of women friends who are open to discussing the intimate details of their sex lives sensitively together, can be very helpful. However, finding such confidantes may or may not be possible in your community. Joining a woman's group that is specifically oriented toward sexual problems, which is led by an experienced female sex therapist, may be an ideal solution, but, again, such programs may not be available in your area. However, more and more reputable sex therapy programs are becoming available.[1] When you work together with other women, it gives you an opportunity to see that you are not alone in your sexual difficulties. You can learn from each other by sharing experiences and by developing more alternatives and solutions to problems than you might have been able to do on your own. And most important, a group of women working together can provide a significant measure of support in the attempt to make changes. Women working closely together and sharing intimately can create a very powerful force.

Some women may find it necessary to change certain aspects of their relationship with their partners in order to become orgasmic. Both people may need to develop skills in communicating or receive help in learning to express feelings more openly. If the man frequently has problems getting or holding an erection, or if he ejaculates almost immediately after intercourse begins, it might be best for the couple to seek sex or marital counseling together. Receiving counseling together is important if the sexual problem is indicative of other problems in the relationship and therefore cannot be treated as an isolated issue or by working with only one partner.

This book and the women's therapy groups are both about liberation in the most basic sense: liberation from the social scripting that prevents women (and men, though perhaps in different ways) from taking control of their lives and expressing themselves as complete and autonomous individuals—free to act the way they feel despite the opinions of others.

Sexual liberation entails acceptance of your own unique sexual responses and sexuality in general, not because it conforms to external standards or solely because it provides pleasure for a partner, but because it is an intimate expression of yourself.

Being sexually liberated means having the freedom to choose—to choose the kind of stimulation that works for you; to choose the sexual activities that are pleasurable for you. It also means being free to choose *not* to do things that fail to meet your needs or values. Being sexually liberated means having in harmony your beliefs, feelings, actions, and desires about your own sexuality.

Sexual liberation is one aspect of personal liberation. Taking control of your life, at the most intimate, personal, and fundamental level—the level of your sexuality—seems to lead to extending control over other areas of life. The women in the groups not only became orgasmic, but, in many cases, found new jobs, terminated unsatisfactory relationships, and initiated new relationships. In general, they became more assertive in having their needs, both sexual and nonsexual, met. They became more self-assured and felt far better about themselves and their bodies.

Once we feel better about ourselves, once we assume that we have rights that deserve respect from others, we are in a position to begin liberating ourselves from the roles society has prescribed. Women's liberation, by freeing women, may in turn free men from their counterpart roles. Such liberation would allow women the freedom to speak, to teach, to be an authority in areas of their own competency. It could thereby free men from having to be experts, allowing them to listen and learn without feeling threatened. Liberation means having the freedom to be strong and caring of others, while still being able to be open and accepting of care from others. Liberation entails being free to be passive and receiving or to be assertive and giving—to be aggressive or nurturing. And most important, being liberated means the freedom to say no, because when you can say no when you want to, you are more free to say yes—and really mean it. Being able to say no makes saying yes a purer pleasure. Being in control of your life means being free to say either.

When you can take control of your life and feel free to be yourself, when you are personally liberated, you lose fear. Feeling secure within yourself diminishes fear of others, of the unknown—fear of that which is unfamiliar or of those who are different. This diminished fear coupled with a sense of self-respect allows for greater respect of others and their rights to be themselves—each being free and self-determined.

Sexual liberation is a beginning.

Notes

Introduction

1. Laumann, Gagnon, Michael, and Michaels (1994) p. 371.
2. Barbach (1974).
3. Masters and Johnson (1970), pp. 295–316
4. Lobitz and LoPiccolo (1972), pp. 267–68.

5. Lobitz and LoPiccolo (1972), pp. 267-68.
6. Hurlbert (1991), pp. 183–90.
7. Nelson (1974), pp. 44–45.
8. Kinsey (1953), p. 146, found there is far greater variety sexually among females than among males.

Chapter 1

1. Personal communication with Dr. Alan Margolis, Ob-Gyn., U.C. Medical Center, San Francisco.
2. Masters and Johnson (1966), p. 133.
3. Kleegman (1959), p. 243, Kaplan (1974), p. 32, and Jorgenson (1973), p. 609.
4. Kaplan (1974), p. 32, and Kinsey (1973), p. 371.
5. Clark and Wallin (1965), p. 134.

6. Ford and Beach (1951), pp. 254–55.
7. Kinsey (1953), p. 384.
8. Mead (1949), pp. 218–23.
9. Masters and Johnson (1966), pp. 191–92.
10. Koedt (1971), p. 312.
11. Anderson, Judith, "Everyone Suffers in the Family," San Francisco *Chronicle*, April 15, 1974, p. 15.
12. Laumann, Gagnon,

Michael, and Michaels (1994), p. 340.

13. O'Connor and Stein (1972), p. 165.

14. Kaplan (1974), p. 71.
15. Cohen and Bartlik (1998), p. 139.
16. Sherfey (1973), p. 165.

Chapter 2

1. Freud (1965), p. 118.
2. Masters and Johnson (1966), pp. 45–67.
3. Huelsman (1976).
4. Kinsey (1953), p. 542.
5. Young (1964), pp. 169–80.
6. Webster (1966), p. 761.
7. Webster (1966), p. 275.
8. Webster (1966), p. 1607.
9. Ford and Beach (1951), p. 266.
10. Ford and Beach (1951), p. 266.
11. Hunt (1974), pp. 155–56.
12. Laumann, Gagnon, Michael, and Michaels (1994), p. 324.

Chapter 4

1. "J" (1969), p. 97.

Chapter 5

1. Masters and Johnson (1966), pp. 56–57.
2. Lowry (1976), chapter titled: "Some Issues in the Histology of the Clitoris."
3. Kaplan (1974), p. 28.
4. Masters and Johnson (1966), p. 191.
5. Lowry (1976), chapter titled: "Some Issues in the Histology of the Clitoris."
6. Kegel (1952), pp. 521–24.
7. Personal communication with Dr. Alan Margolis, Ob-Gyn., U.C. Medical Center, San Francisco.
8. Kaplan (1974), p. 441.
9. Netter (1965), p. 3.
10. Masters and Johnson (1966), p. 45.
11. Kaplan (1974), p. 72.
12. Kinsey (1953), p. 163.
13. Masters and Johnson (1966), pp. 27–170.
14. Masters and Johnson (1966), p. 66.
15. Kaplan (1974), pp. 106–8.
16. Kinsey (1973), p. 375.

17. Bergler and Kroger (1954), p. 82.
18. Masters and Johnson (1966), p. 65.

Chapter 6

1. Kinsey (1953), pp. 668–69.
2. Kaplan (1974), p. 63.
3. Fisher (1973), p. 280.
4. Kinsey (1953), pp. 670–72
5. Hunt (1974), p. 24.
6. Schmidt and Sigusch (1973), pp. 117–44.
7. Hunt (1974), pp. 90–93; p. 332.
8. *Cabin Fever, The Voyeur,* and *The Hottest Bid* can be

Chapter 7

1. Kinsey (1953), p. 133.
2. Kinsey (1953), p. 133.
3. Kinsey (1953), p. 142.
4. Kinsey (1953), p. 132.
5. Kinsey (1953), p. 172.
6. Kinsey (1953), pp. 386–91.
7. Masters and Johnson (1966), p. 133; p. 313.
8. Kinsey (1953), p. 171.
9. Sherfey (1966), p. 144.
10. Laumann, Gagnon, Michael, and Michaels (1994), p. 86.
11. Gordon (1968), pp. 21–26.
12. Gordon (1968), p. 30.

19. Personal communication with Dr. Len Laskow, Ob-Gyn., U.C. Medical Center, San Francisco.

purchased by calling 310-589-5849. *What Women Want* and *More of What Women Want* are sexually explicit videos and can be ordered by calling 818-508-1296.

9. Kinsey (1953), p. 164.
10. Kaplan (1974), pp. 88–89.
11. Kaplan (1974), p. 90.

13. Ford and Beach (1951), p. 155.
14. Kinsey (1953), p. 169.
15. Mead (1949), p. 218.
16. Greenberg (1973), p. 48.
17. Young (1964), p. 170.
18. Kinsey (1953), p. 169.
19. Landis (1940), p. 210.
20. Laumann, Gagnon, Michael, and Michaels (1994), p. 82.
21. Kinsey (1953), p. 170.
22. Hunt (1974), p. 76.
23. Kinsey (1953), p. 142.
24. Kinsey (1953), p. 132.

Chapter 8

1. The Panasonic vibrator is particularly well liked. Vibrators can be obtained through:

Good Vibrations
1210 Valencia St.
San Francisco, Ca.
800-289-8423

Chapter 9

1. Exercises outlined in Rosenberg's *Total Orgasm* have been found beneficial by many women.

2. Martin and Lyon (1972), p. 88.
3. Kinsey (1953), p. 161.

Chapter 10

1. Koedt (1971), pp. 311–20, Masters and Johnson (1966), p. 66, Sherfey (1966), p. 142, and Kaplan (1974), p. 377.

2. Wallach (1973), p. 47.
3. Hunt (1974), p. 20.
4. Moulton (1973), p. 245.

Chapter 12

1. *Lover's Massage* can be ordered by calling 818-508-1296.
2. Masters and Johnson (1970), pp. 71–75.

3. Rosenberg (1973), pp. 170–71.
4. Gebhard (1966), p. 95.

Chapter 13

1. Laumann, Gagnon, Michael, and Michaels (1994), p. 105.
2. Kelly, p. 10.

3. Laumann, Gagnon, Michael, and Michaels (1994), p. 130.
4. Shulman (1971), pp. 301–2.

Chapter 14

1. Masters and Johnson (1966), pp. 156–57.

2. Solberg, Butler, and Wagner (1973), p. 1098.

3. Masters and Johnson (1966), p. 143.
4. Solberg, Butler, and Wagner (1973), p. 1102.
5. White (1982), p. 429, and Perkins (1982), p. 189.
6. Masters and Johnson (1966), p. 136, and Solberg, Butler, and Wagner (1973), p. 1102.
7. Masters and Johnson (1966), p. 146.
8. Masters and Johnson (1966), p. 159.
9. Sherfey (1972), p. 101.
10. Masters and Johnson (1966), p. 149.
11. Solberg, Butler, and Wagner (1973), p. 1100.
12. Solberg, Butler, and Wagner (1973), p. 1101.
13. Masters and Johnson (1966), p. 168.
14. Israel and Rubin (1967), p. 11.
15. Solberg, Butler, and Wagner (1973), p. 1102.
16. Israel and Rubin (1967), p. 10.
17. Solberg, Butler, and Wagner (1973), p. 1100.
18. Masters and Johnson (1966), p. 160.
19. Personal communication with Dr. Alan Margolis, Ob-Gyn., U.C. Medical Center, San Francisco.
20. Masters and Johnson (1966), p. 167.
21. Israel and Rubin (1967), p. 13.
22. Sherfey (1972), p. 101.
23. Masters and Johnson (1966), p. 163.
24. Brecher (1966), p. 90.
25. Pomeroy (1974), p. 33.
26. Brecher (1966), p. 92.
27. Masters and Johnson (1966), pp. 240–41.

Chapter 15
1. Book Collective (1971), pp. 106–37.
2. Semler (1995), p. 225.

Chapter 16
1. Ribble (1944), pp. 621–51.
2. Shulman (1971), p. 293.
3. Landis (1940), p. 210.
4. Kinsey (1953), p. 172.

Chapter 17

1. For information regarding reputable sex therapists or sex therapy programs in your area, write or call:

American Association of Marriage and Family Counselors
(800) 374-2638

American Association of Sex Educators and Counselors
P.O. Box 238
Mt. Vernon, IA 52314
319-895-8407

Sex Information and Education Council of the U.S.
130 W. 42nd St.
Suite 2500
New York, N.Y. 10036
212-819-9770

Your local American Medical Association or Planned Parenthood offices may also have listings of programs in your area.

Bibliography

Abbott, Sidney and Love, Barbara. *Sappho Was a Right-On Woman: A Liberated View of Lesbianism*. New York: Stein & Day, 1972.

Bach, George and Wyden, Peter. *The Intimate Enemy: How to Fight Fair in Love and Marriage*. New York: Avon Books, 1968.

Barbach, Lonnie G. "Group Treatment of Pre-Orgasmic Women," *Journal of Sex and Marital Therapy*, v. 1, no. 2, 1974.

Barbach, Lonnie G. *For Each Other: Sharing Sexual Intimacy*. New York: Anchor Press, Doubleday, 1982 and New York: Signet, New American Library, 1982.

Barbach Lonnie G., Ed. *Pleasures: Women Write Erotica*. New York: HarperCollins, 1984.

Barbach, Lonnie G., Ed. *Erotic Interludes: Tales Told by Women*. New York: Dutton, 1995.

Barbach, Lonnie G., Ed. *The Erotic Edge: 22 Erotic Stories for Couples*. New York: Dutton, 1994.

Barbach, Lonnie G. *Turn Ons: Pleasing Yourself While You Please Your Lover*. New York: Dutton, 1997.

Barbach, Lonnie G., Ed. *Seductions: Tales of Erotic Persuasion*. New York: Dutton, 1999.

Barbach, Lonnie G. *The Pause: Positive Approaches to Perimenopause and Menopause*. New York: Dutton, 2000.

Barbach, Lonnie G. *Women Discover Orgasm: A Therapist's Guide to a New Treatment Approach*. Houston (Electronic Version): TLG Media Inc., 2000.

Barbach, Lonnie G. and Geisinger, David. *Going the Distance: Finding and Keeping Lifelong Love*. New York: Doubleday, 1991.

Barbach, Lonnie G. and Levine, Linda. *Shared Intimacies: Women's Sexual Experiences*. Gretna, LA (Electronic Version): Wellness Institute, Inc., 2000.

Belliveau, Fred and Richter, Lin. *Understanding Human Sexual Inadequacy*. Boston: Little, Brown & Co., 1970.

Bergler, E. and Kroger, W. S. *Kinsey's Myth of Female Sexuality*. New York: Grune & Stratton, 1954.

The Boston Women's Health Book Collective. *Our Bodies, Ourselves: A Book By and For Women*. New York: Simon & Schuster, 1971, 1973.

Brecher, Ruth and Brecher, Edward, Eds. *An Analysis of Human Sexual Response*. New York: Signet, New American Library, 1966.

Brecher, Ruth and Brecher, Edward. "Sex During and After Pregnancy," *An Analysis of Human Sexual Response*. Brecher, Ruth and Brecher, Edward, Eds. New York: Signet, New American Library, 1966, pp. 88–95.

Clark, Alexander L. and Wallin, Paul. "Women's Sexual Responsiveness and the Duration and Quality of their Marriages," *American Journal of Sociology*, v. 71, 1965, pp. 187–96.

Cleland, John. *Fanny Hill: Memoirs of a Woman of Pleasure*. North Hollywood: Brandon House, 1963.

Clifford, Ruth. Unpublished Doctoral Thesis on Masturbation, Stonybrook, 1973.

Cohen, A. J. and Bartlik, B. "Ginkgo biloba for antidepressant-induced sexual dysfunction," *Journal of Sex and Marital Therapy*, v. 24, no. 2, 1998, pp. 139–43.

Dodson, Betty. *Sex For One: The Joy of Selfloving*. New York: Crown Publishers, Inc., 1996.

Downing, George. *The Massage Book*. New York: Random House, and Berkeley: The Bookworks, 1972.

Fisher, Seymour. *The Female Orgasm*. New York: Basic Books, Inc., 1973.

Ford, Clellans and Beach, Frank A. *Patterns of Sexual Behavior*. New York: Harper & Row, 1951.

Frankfort, Ellen. *Vaginal Politics*. New York: Bantam Books, National General Co., 1972.

Freud, Sigmund, Trans. and Ed. by Strachey, James. *New Introductory Lectures on Psychoanalysis*. New York: W. W. Norton & Co., Inc., 1965

Friday, Nancy. *Forbidden Flowers*. New York: Pocket Books, 1993.

Friday, Nancy. *My Secret Garden: Women's Sexual Fantasies*. New York: Pocket Books, 1973.

Gebhard, P. H. "Factors in Marital Orgasm," *The Journal of Social Issues*, v. 22, 1966, pp. 88–95.

Gornick, Vivian and Moran, Barbara K., Eds. *Woman in Sexist Society: Studies in Power and Powerlessness*. New York: Signet, New American Library, 1971.

Gravelle, Karen, Gravelle, Jennifer, and Palen, Debbie. *The Period Book*. New York: Walker and Company, 1996.

Greenberg, Jerold S. and Archambault, Francis X. "Masturbation, Self-Esteem and Other Variables," *Journal of Sex Research*, v. 9, no. 1, 1973, pp. 41–51.

Harris, Robie. *It's Perfectly Normal: Changing Bodies, Growing Up, Sex and Sexual Health*. Cambridge, Mass., Candlewick Press, 1996.

Herschberger, Ruth. *Adam's Rib*. New York: Pellegrini and Cudahy, 1948.

Hite, Shere. *The Hite Report: A Nationwide Study of Female Sexuality*. New York: Dell Publishing Co., 1977.

Huelsman, Ben R. "An Anthropological View of Clitoral and Other Female Genital Mutilations," *The Clitoris*. Lowry, Thomas and Lowry, Thea S., Eds. St. Louis: Warren H. Green Publishers, 1976.

Hunt, Morton. "Sexual Behavior in the 1970's," *Playboy*, October 1973.

Hunt, Morton. *Sexual Behavior in the 1970's*. Chicago: Playboy Press, 1974.

Hurlbert, D. F. "The role of assertiveness in female sexuality: a comparative study between sexually assertive and sexually nonassertive women," *The Journal of Sex and Marital Therapy*, v. 17, no. 3, 1991, pp. 183–90.

Israel, Leon and Rubin, Isadore. *Sexual Relations During Pregnancy and the Post-Delivery Period*. New York: SIECUS Publications, 1967.

"J." *The Sensuous Woman*. New York: Dell Publishing Co., 1969.

Jukes, Mavis and Tilley, Debbie, Illus., *Growing Up: It's a Girl Thing*. New York: Knopf, 1998.

Kaplan, Helen Singer. *The New Sex Therapy*. New York: Brunner/Mazel, 1974.

Kegel, A. H. "Sexual Functions of the Pubococcygeus Muscle," *Western Journal of Surgery*, v. 60, no. 10, 1952, pp. 521–24.

Kelly, Kathy. "Radical Sex Manual," Unpublished Paper.

Kinsey, Alfred C., Pomeroy, Wardell B., Martin, Clyde E., and Gebhard, Paul H. *Sexual Behavior in the Human Female*. New York: Pocket Books, Simon & Schuster, 1953.

Kleegman, Sophia. "Frigidity in Women," *Quarterly Review of Surgery, Obstetrics and Gynecology*, v. 16, 1959, pp. 243–48.

Koedt, Ann. "The Myth of the Vaginal Orgasm," *Liberation Now*. Babcox, Deborah and Belkin, Madeline, Eds. New York: Dell Publishing Co., 1971, pp. 311–20.

Levine, Linda and Barbach, Lonnie G. *The Intimate Male: Candid Discussions about Women, Sex, and Relationships*. Gretna, LA (Electronic Version): Wellness Institute, Inc., 2000.

Lobitz, W. Charles and LoPiccolo, Joseph. "New Methods in the Behavioral Treatment of Sexual Dysfunction," *Journal of Behavior Therapy and Experimental Psychiatry*, v. 3, 1972, pp. 265–71.

Lowry, Thomas P. "Some Issues in the Histology of the Clitoris," *The Clitoris*. Lowry, Thomas P. and Lowry, Thea S., Eds. St. Louis: Warren H. Green Publishers, 1976.

Lowry, Thomas P. and Lowry, Thea, S., Eds. *The Clitoris*. St. Louis: Warren H. Green Publishers, 1976.

Lydon, Susan. "The Politics of Orgasm," *Sisterhood Is Powerful*. Morgan, Robin, Ed. New York: Vintage Books, Random House, 1970, pp. 197–204.

Madaras, Lynda, Saavedra, Dane, and Lopez, Ralph. *The What's Happening to My Body? Book for Boys*. New York: Newmarket Press, 1987.

Martin, Del and Lyon, Phillis. *Lesbian Woman*. New York: Bantam Books, National General Co., 1972.

Masters, William H. and Johnson, Virginia E. *Human Sexual Response*. Boston: Little, Brown & Co., 1966.

Masters, William H. and Johnson, Virginia E. *Human Sexual Inadequacy*. Boston: Little, Brown & Co., 1970.

Mead, Margaret. *Male and Female: A Study of the Sexes in a Changing World*. New York: Laurel Editions, Dell Publishing Co., 1949.

Moulton, Ruth. "A Survey and Reevaluation of the Concept of Penis Envy," *Psychoanalysis and Women*. Miller, Jean Baker, Ed. Baltimore: Penguin Books, Inc., 1973, pp. 239–58.

Nelson, Arvalea. "Personality Attributes of Female Orgasmic Consistency (or, Romance Makes You Frigid)," Unpublished M.A. Thesis for University of California, Berkeley, 1974.

Netter, Frank H. *The CIBA Collection of Medical Illustrations*, v. 2, Summit, New Jersey: CIBA Corporation, 1954, 1965.

O'Connor, John F. and Stern, Lenore O. "Results of Treatment in Functional Sexual Disorders," *New York Journal of Medicine*, v. 72, no. 15, 1972, pp. 127–34.

Otto, Herbert A. and Otto, Roberta. *Total Sex*. New York: Signet, New American Library, 1972.

The Pearl. New York: Grove Press, 1967.

Penner, Clifford and Penner, Joyce. *The Gift of Sex: A Christian Guide to Sexual Fulfillment*. Word: Word Books, 1981.

Perkins, R. P. "Sexuality in Pregnancy: What Determines Behavior?" *Obstetrics and Gynecology*, v. 59, no. 2, 1982, pp. 189–98.

Pomeroy, Wardell. *Boys and Sex*. New York: Dell Publishing Co., 1968.

Pomeroy, Wardell. *Girls and Sex*. New York: Dell Publishing Co., 1969.

Pomeroy, Wardell. *Dr. Kinsey and the Institute for Sex Research*. New York: Signet, New American Library, 1973.

Pomeroy, Wardell. *Your Child and Sex: A Guide to Parents*. New York: Delacorte Press, 1974.

Ribble, M. "The Infantile Experience in Relation to Personality

Development," *Personality and the Behavior Disorders*. Hunt, J. McV., Ed. New York: Ronald Press, 1944, pp. 621–51.

Rosenberg, Jack Lee. *Total Orgasm*. New York: Random House, and Berkeley: The Bookworks, 1973.

Rubin, I. "Sex After Forty—and After Seventy," *An Analysis of Human Sexual Response*. Brecher, Ruth and Brecher, Edward, Eds. New York: Signet, New American Library, 1966, pp. 251–66.

Rush, Ann Kent. *Getting Clear*. New York: Random House, and Berkeley: The Bookworks, 1973.

Schmidt, Gunter and Sigusch, Volkmar. "Women's Sexual Arousal," *Contemporary Sexual Behavior: Critical Issues in the 1970's*. Zubin, Joseph and Money, John, Eds. American Psychopathological Association Proceedings, 61st, 1971. Baltimore: The Johns Hopkins University Press, 1973.

Semler, Tracy Chutorian. *All About Eve: The Complete Guide to Women's Health and Well-Being*. New York: Harper Collins, 1995.

Sherfey, Mary Jane. *The Nature and Evolution of Female Sexuality*. New York: Vintage Books, Random House, 1966, 1972.

Sherfey, Mary Jane. "On the Nature of Female Sexuality," *Psychoanalysis and Women*. Miller, Jean Baker, Ed. Baltimore: Penguin Books, Inc., 1973, pp. 135–54.

Sherfey, Mary Jane. "A Theory on Female Sexuality," *Sisterhood Is Powerful*. Morgan, Robin, Ed. New York: Vintage Books, Random House, 1970, pp. 220–29.

Shulman, Alix. "Organs and Orgasms," *Woman in Sexist Society*. Gornick, Vivian and Moran, Barbara K., Eds. New York: Signet, New American Library, 1971, pp. 292–303.

Solberg, Don A., Butler, Julius, and Wagner, Nathaniel N. "Sexual Behavior and Pregnancy," *The New England Journal of Medicine*, v. 288, no. 21, May 24, 1973, pp. 1098–103.

Wallace, Doug and Barbach, Lonnie. "Pre-Orgasmic Group Treatment," *Journal of Sex and Marital Therapy*, v. 1, no. 2, 1975.

Wallach, Leah. "Vaginal vs. Clitoral Orgasm," *Forum*, v. 2, no. 7, September 1973, pp. 44–47.

Wallin, Paul and Clark, Alexander L. "A Study of Orgasm as a Condition of Woman's Enjoyment of Coitus in the Middle Years of Marriage," *Human Biology*, v. 35, May 1963, pp. 131–39.

Webster, *New World Dictionary*. College Edition. New York: The World Publishing Company, 1966.

White, S. E. and Reamy, K. "Sex and Pregnancy: A Review," *Archives of Sexual Behavior*, v. 11, no. 5, 1982, pp. 429–44.

Young, Wayland. *Eros Denied*. New York: Grove Press, Inc., 1964.

Zilbergeld, Bernie. *The New Male Sexuality*. New York: Bantam Books, 1999.

Index